Dental Caries: Impact on Human Health

First Edition

Dr. Dinesh. M.D., M.Sc., Ph.D.
Assistant Professor
Department of Microbiology,
Nehru Arts and Science College (Autonomous)
(NASC), Thirumalayampalayam, Coimbatore, Tamil Nadu.
(Affiliated to Bharathiar University).

Dr. Thulasi Sivaraman, M.Phil., Ph.D.
Assistant Professor
Department of Microbiology,
Nehru Arts and Science College (Autonomous)
(NASC), Thirumalayampalayam, Coimbatore, Tamil Nadu.
(Affiliated to Bharathiar University).

Thushara James, M.Sc. MPhil.
Research Scholar (Ph.D.)
PG & Research Department of Aquaculture Microbiology
MES Ponnani College, Ponnani, (Calicut University)
Malappuram, Kerala.

FoxGales Publication

Proud Imprint of Noverse Foundation
Vadakkenchery, Palakkad, Kerala - 678683

Website: www.foxgalespublication.com

Email id: foxgalespublication@gmail.com

LinkedIn: www.linkedin.com/company/foxgalespublication

Instagram: foxgalespublication

Facebook: FoxGales Publication

Author – Dr. M.D. Dinesh
Co-Auhtor – Dr. Thulasi Sivaraman, Thushara James
Book Title: *Dental Caries*
ISBN: 978-81-978636-5-3

Processed and printed in India

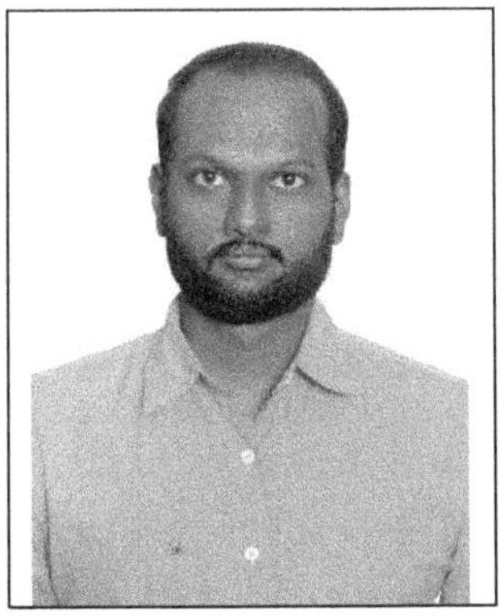

Dr. M.D. Dinesh possesses approximately 10 years of teaching experience in undergraduate and postgraduate classes. He earned an M.Sc. and Ph.D. in Microbiology with a specialization in Immunology and Immuno-technology from Bharathiar University, Coimbatore. Currently, he serves as an Assistant Professor in the Department of Microbiology at Nehru Arts and Science College (Autonomous), Coimbatore. Dr. Dinesh has authored 35 research papers in various peer-reviewed journals of international repute. His primary research areas include Dental Cariology, Anti-venom studies (Antidote and Antibody Development), and Aquaculture Microbiology. Additionally, he has contributed chapters to numerous books and supervised research for both M. Phil. and Ph.D. candidates at Bharathiar University. Recognized for his contributions, Dr. Dinesh has received grants for Minor Projects from the Department of Science and Technology, Government of India. He holds memberships in the Association of Microbiologist India (AMI), Indian Science Congress (ICS), and the American Society for Microbiology (ASM).

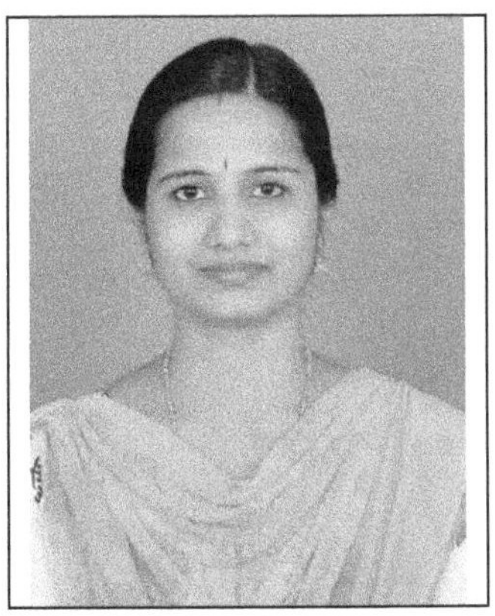

Dr. Thulasi Sivaraman has about 6 years of Teaching experience of undergraduate post graduate classes. She did her M.Sc., M. Phil., and Ph.D. studies in Microbiology at Bharathiar University in Coimbatore, with a focus on Medical Microbiology. She is currently employed as an Assistant Professor in the Nehru Arts and Science College (autonomous) Microbiology Department in Coimbatore. She has had research papers published 10 research articles in internationally recognized peer-reviewed Journals. Anti-venom research is one of the preliminary fields of study. Research supervisor at Bharathiar University for Ph.D. and M.Phil. programs. Received Grants (Minor project) from Department of Science and Technology, Government of India. She holds memberships in the Association of Microbiologist India (AMI), Indian Science Congress (ICS), and the American Society for Microbiology (ASM).

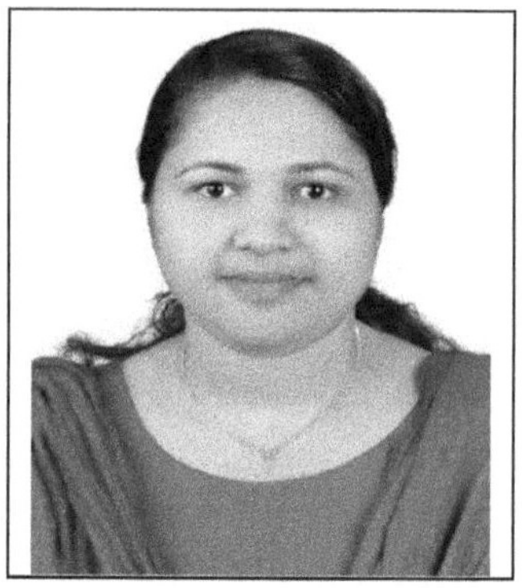

Thushara James is an active research scholar in the PG and Research Department of Aquaculture and Microbiology, MES Ponnani College (Affiliated with Calicut University) Ponnani, Malappuram, Kerala. She did her M.Sc. and M.Phil. in Microbiology at Bharathiar University in Coimbatore, with an emphasis on Immunology and Immunotechnology. She has had research papers published in a number of internationally recognized peer-reviewed Journals. Studies on Anti-venom and Aquaculture Microbiology are important fields of study. She has also written several book chapters. She has presented her research ideas at National and International conferences. She had won the NSDCA Vocational Educational Council's International Conference Best Presenter Award. She is a member of both the American Society for Microbiology and the Association of Microbiologists of India (AMI).

PREFACE

Cariology is a branch of dental science that focuses on the investigation of microbial tooth decay. The branch also includes tooth decay or injury to the tooth's tissue. The prevention of oral diseases is another goal of modern science. The oral cavity is a bizarre place for both pathogenic and normal flora germs to live. Microorganisms have a better chance of surviving when certain conditions are met, such as saliva, pH, etc. An individual's mouth cavity is entirely sterile at birth, but germs begin to colonize it after the very first feeding. Teeth and their surrounding tissues are generally prone to numerous disorders. Teeth decay or cavities are the most frequent noncommunicable disease affecting people of all ages globally.

Even when human life on Earth ends, its incurable diseases continue to exist. Prevention tactics are preferable to eradication in order to get out of this predicament. There are numerous variable elements that affect the persistence of dental carriers, such as food habits, social and economic issues. Severe dental caries can lead to pain, infection, and even the need to extraction of teeth. It also has an adverse effect on overall health. The best way to deal with the circumstances is to be aware of the importance of dental hygiene. Governmental organizations connected to dentistry societies worldwide offer numerous public awareness campaigns. In India as well, data collection and statistical updating are necessary. The development of dental caries and poor oral hygiene will have an adverse effect on human health, increasing the risk of endocarditis, strokes, pregnancy-related difficulties, and diabetes mellitus.

Written for a wide range of college students, including science grads and middle schoolers, researchers, and anybody interested in learning more about dental caries, this book covers the fundamentals of dental caries, oral hygiene, and other oral issues. The subject matter has been presented clearly, organized neatly, and abundantly illustrated. Each chapter ends with a list of references and internet resources to help the reader find both classic and contemporary literature. At the end of the book, there is an arrangement of abbreviations. The primary illustrations are taken from books and journals that are typical. Every figure has a legend that properly acknowledges its source. The original version of 'X-Checker' was used to check each chapter for plagiarism, and reduced the rate up to 20%.

We author also thankful to our publisher, finally we are grateful to thank our family members, Mr. Ajish Jhon and Aneesh. S, and Mrs. Megha Das., for inspiring us in proceeding from thoughts to points.

Dr. Dinesh. M.D., Dr. Thulasi Sivaraman., Thushara James.

Part- I Microbiology of Dental Diseases **Page No**

CHAPTER

1

Dental Caries

HIGHLIGHTS

- Cariologists are dentists who specialize in cariology, the study of the elements that lead to the development of dental caries.
- The French physician Pierre Fauchard, called the "Father of Dentistry."
- Dental caries, sometimes referred to as tooth decay or a cavity, is an illness brought on by certain bacteria that exist in the mouths of humans.
- Human teeth are colonized by both normal and harmful bacteria in the oral cavity from birth. Two of the main bacteria that cause dental caries are *Streptococcus mutans* and *Streptococcus mitis*.
- There are several treatment options available to prevent dental caries, including the use of antibiotics, vaccinations, herbal remedies, etc.

Cariology is the branch of Dentistry and Dental medicine that focuses on the study of Dental caries, commonly known as tooth decay or cavities. It involves the investigation of the causes, development, prevention, and treatment of dental caries. The goal of cariology is to understand the mechanisms of tooth decay and develop effective strategies for preventing and treating dental caries. This may involve promoting good oral hygiene practices, educating individuals about the impact of diet on oral health, and developing new technologies and materials to prevent and repair tooth damage. Cariologists study the various factors that contribute to the formation of cavities, including the role of bacteria, the composition of saliva, dietary habits, and oral hygiene practices. Cariology's history dates back to the prehistoric era, when individuals first noticed and encountered tooth rot. Evidence from the Ancient Civilizations shows that dental issues, including tooth decay, were known to exist in ancient societies including Egypt, Greece, and Rome. Toothpaste-like substances and other medicines were used to clean teeth and gums. In the Middle Ages, toothaches and other oral health disorders were frequently treated with a combination of superstition and poor medical understanding. Dental hygiene measures were also sometimes inadequate.

The 17th century saw considerable awareness of the theory that tiny organisms produced dental cavities. The "father of modern dentistry," Pierre Fauchard, a French physician, made important advances in dental science with his book "Le Chirurgien Dentiste" (The Surgeon Dentist). The 18th century saw advances in our knowledge of dental anatomy and function. Although they were still in their infancy, advancements in dental tools and methods began to appear. The 19th century saw a growing body of evidence linking sugar consumption to tooth decay, and developments in dental education and the formation of dental societies furthered the field's understanding of dentistry. The 20th century Water fluoridation programs were put into place as a result of the finding that fluoride can reduce tooth decay. The knowledge of oral microbiology and how bacteria, especially *Streptococcus mutans*, contribute to tooth decay has grown. Cavity therapy has been enhanced by developments in restorative dentistry, such as the creation of dental materials like composite resins. From the late 20th century to now ongoing investigation of the components causing dental caries.

Oral and Dental Health have improved enormously over the last century in the urbanized countries, but the prevalence of dental caries in the developing countries like India remains a considerable clinical problem. At present various caries defensive strategies are in use like oral health education, chemical and mechanical control of plaque, use of fluoride and its application of pit and fissure sealants etc. A lot of these approaches can be broadly effective and profitable. However behavioural or cultural barriers to their use encompass constant the epidemic of dental disease in the mouths of many people on a global level. Dental caries is an infectious disease of the teeth that results in localized dissolution and destruction of the calcified tissues. It is considered to be a disease of civilized society, related to lifestyle factors, but heredity also plays a role. Dental caries is a multifactorial human disease that has widely affected many populations all over the world. This is caused by accumulation of biofilm on tooth surface (Marsh *et al*., 2006). Manifestations of the disease occur when there is an imbalance between the biofilm and the host due to changes in biofilm matrix pH caused by diet, microorganisms, or salivary flow and their components (Kajfasz *et al*., 2010).

Dental plaque is a general term for the diverse microbial community (predominantly bacteria) found on the tooth surface, embedded in a matrix of polymers of bacterial and salivary origin. Dental caries will not occur if the oral cavity is free of bacteria. These bacteria are organized into a material known as dental plaque which is yellowish coloured film on the surface of the teeth. Of the many types of bacteria in the mouth, the most caries active appear to be *Streptococcus mutans, Streptococcus mitis,* Lactobacillus sp., Veillonella sp. and Actinomyces sp. These bacteria can be transferred from mother to child and are present at varying levels in all human mouths. A variety of carbohydrates provide substrates for these organisms to grow on and the waste products of their metabolism - acids - initiate the tooth decay process by dissolving tooth enamel. These bacteria produce acid that destroys tooth enamel and results in cavities on its surface. The principle causative agent of dental caries is a group of Streptococcal species collectively referred to as the mutans streptococci, of which *Streptococcus mutans* and *Streptococcus mitis* are the most important agents of human dental caries.

Antibiotics are constantly in use for treating dental caries, it has been used in aspire of eradication or inhibition of biofilm in the oral cavity. Penicillin, methicillin, ampicillin, erythromycin, cephalothin, chlorhexidine digluconate and many other antibiotics have been reported to effectively prevent dental caries more than ever viridians streptococci in humans and animals. These antibiotics are never used clinically because of many adverse effects such as hypersensitivity reactions, supra infections and teeth staining. A high concentration of antibiotics causes coagulation of the intracellular constituents. As a result, the cytoplasm becomes congealed, with a resulting reduction in leakage (In-detail Chapter - 15). The latest approach for combating dental caries is through the development of an efficient vaccine that is well suited for public health applications especially in environments that do not lend themselves to regular health care (In-detail Chapter - 16). This book provides a comprehensive overview of dental caries, the role microbes play in its creation, and the effects caries has on human health.

References

Dinesh, M.D., A. Shaheena, K.K. Abdul Bari, Neethu George and Meenatchisundaram, S (2016). Preliminary screening of Anticariogenic properties of selected medicinal plants against Streptococcal dental caries. Int.J.Curr.Microbiol.App.Sci.5(1): 699-705.

Kajfasz, J. K. J. Abranches., A.R. Martinez., P.L. Rosalen., A.M. Derr., R.G. Quivey and J.A. Lemos. 2010. Two Spx proteins modulate stress tolerance, survival, and virulence in *Streptococcus mutans*. *J Bacteriol.* **192:** 2546–2556.

Loesche, W. J. 1986. Role of *Streptococcus mutans* in human dental decay. *Microbiol. Rev.* **50:** 353-380.

M Balakrishnan, R S Simmonds, J R Tagg. Dental caries is a preventable infectious disease. (2000). Aust Dent J. 2000 Dec;45(4):235-45. doi: 10.1111/j.1834-7819. 2000.tb00257.

Madhavi Wig, Adarsh Kumar, Manjunath Bhadravathi Chaluvaiah, Vipul Yadav, Mansi Mendiratta and Amit Aggarwal. Dental caries vaccine: An overview. (2021). International Journal of Applied Dental Sciences. IJADS 2021; 7(2): 461-465.

Marsh, P.D. 2006. Dental plaque as a biofilm and a microbial community implication for health and disease. *BMC Oral Health. 6 Suppl.* **1:** 14.

Mohammad Khursheed Alam, Huda Abutayyem, Bushra Kanwal, and Maher A. L. Shayeb. Future of Orthodontics—A Systematic Review and Meta-Analysis on the Emerging Trends in This Field. J Clin Med. 2023 Jan; 12(2): 532. doi: 10.3390/jcm12020532.

Naseem Shah. Oral and dental diseases: Causes, prevention and treatment strategies. Oral and dental diseases: Causes, prevention and treatment strategies. NCMH Background Papers· Burden of Disease in India. 1-24.

Nélio Veiga, Ricardo Figueiredo, Patrícia Correia, Pedro Lopes, Patrícia Couto, and Gustavo Vicentis Oliveira Fernandes. Methods of Primary Clinical Prevention of Dental Caries in the Adult Patient: An Integrative Review. Healthcare (Basel). 2023 Jun; 11(11): 1635. doi: 10.3390/healthcare11111635.

Oleksandr Grytsai, Iuliia Myrgorodska, Stéphane Rocchi, Cyril Ronco, Rachid Benhida. Biguanides drugs: Past success stories and promising future for drug discovery. European Journal of Medicinal Chemistry.

Philip D Marsh. Dental plaque as a biofilm and a microbial community – implications for health and disease. BMC Oral Health. 2006; 6(Suppl 1): S14. doi: 10.1186/1472-6831-6-S1-S14.

Sourabh Badjatia, Rini G Badjatia, K Thanveer, and Ajith CG Krishnan. Effects of Fluoride Varnish on *Streptococcus mutans* Count in Saliva. (2017). Int J Clin Pediatr Dent. 2017 Jan-Mar; 10(1): 62–66.

Yoon Lee. Diagnosis and Prevention Strategies for Dental Caries. J Lifestyle Med. 2013 Sep; 3(2): 107–109.

HIGHLIGHTES

- Oral health, the most prevalent noncommunicable diseases (NCDs) that impact people at any stage of life are oral disorders.
- People with weakened immune systems, the elderly, and children may be more vulnerable to a variety of oral health conditions.
- Oral diseases are more common due to a number of variables, including dietary habits, specific chemical interaction, alcohol intake, chronic stress, and diabetes.
- Research has demonstrated that adopting healthy food and dental practices is essential to achieving and maintaining overall physical and mental well-being throughout life.

CHAPTER 2

Oral and Dental Hygiene

Maintaining good oral and dental hygiene can help you keep your teeth as you age by preventing gum disease, tooth decay, and bad breath. Achieving and sustaining general physical and mental well-being throughout life has been shown to depend on developing appropriate dental hygiene and eating habits. Speech, diet, nutrition, appearance, and interpersonal relationships can all be impacted by our oral health, which can also have an impact on our physical and mental wellbeing. Furthermore, oral diseases have the potential to impact other parts of the body and play a role in some secondary disorders. WHO defines oral health as "a state of being free from chronic mouth and facial pain, oral and throat cancer, oral infection and sores, periodontal (gum) disease, tooth decay, tooth loss, and other diseases and disorders that limit an individual's capacity in biting, chewing, smiling, speaking, and psychosocial wellbeing."

2.1. Tooth and its structure and Function

The human body's teeth are vital organs that are vital to both general oral health and the digestive process. These are specialized mechanisms designed to break up food particles into smaller, more palatable pieces by biting, ripping, and grinding food. The anatomy of teeth is made up of several parts, each of which has a distinct purpose (Table- 1)

Table- 1 Parts of Teeth and its Functions

S.l No	Parts	Functions
1.	Crown	The visible portion of the human body covered in enamel, the toughest material, is the crown. Enamel, the toughest material in the human body, covers it and shields the tooth from damage.
2.	Root	The section of the tooth implanted in the jawbone below the gum line is called the root. It offers stability and anchoring for the teeth.
3.	Enamel	The outermost layer of the crown is called enamel, and it is mostly made of hydroxyapatite minerals. It shields the tooth from external influences and deterioration because of its high mineralization.
4.	Dentin	Beneath the enamel lies the dentin, a hard tissue that comprises most of the tooth's structure. Though not as durable as enamel, it is nevertheless rather strong.
5.	Pulp	The pulp, which extends into the roots from the middle of the crown, is the tooth's innermost layer. It is made up of connective tissue, blood vessels, and nerves. In addition to providing nutrition to the tooth during its growth, the pulp is the tooth's primary pain and temperature sense.
6.	Cementum	The hard tissue known as cementum surrounds the tooth's roots and aids in holding it firmly in place in the jawbone. Though not as strong as enamel, it is essential for the stability of teeth.
7.	Periodontal Ligament (PDL)	Connecting the tooth to the surrounding bone, the PDL is a fibrous tissue that envelops the tooth's roots. By serving as a cushion, it protects the tooth from the forces of biting and chewing.
8.	**Gingiva (Gums)**	Encircling the teeth are the gums, which shield the supporting tissues. The stability of teeth depends on healthy gums.
9.	Alveolar bone	The area of the jawbone that encircles and sustains the tooth roots is called the alveolar bone. It is essential for preserving the stability and location of the teeth.

Figure – 1 Structure of Tooth and its Parts

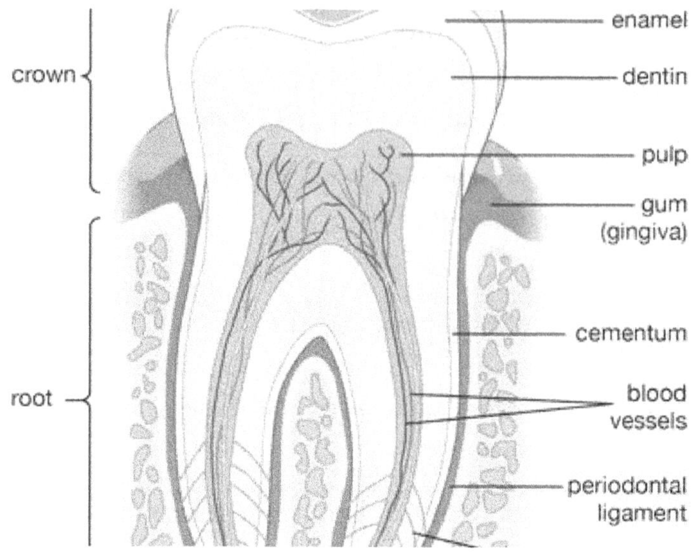

2.2. Importance of Oral Health

Oral diseases are the most common noncommunicable diseases (NCDs) and affect people throughout their lifetime, causing pain, discomfort, disfigurement and even death. The Global Burden of Disease Study 2016 estimated that oral diseases affected half of the world's population (3.58 billion people) with dental caries (tooth decay) in permanent teeth being the most prevalent condition assessed. Globally, it is estimated that 2.4 billion people suffer from caries of permanent teeth and 486 million children suffer from caries of primary teeth. Severe periodontal (gum) disease, which may result in tooth loss, was estimated to be the 11th most prevalent disease globally. Oral hygiene to be carried out on a regular basis to enable prevention of dental disease and bad breath. The most common types of dental disease are tooth decay (cavities, dental caries) and gum diseases, including gingivitis, and periodontitis (Dhage and Pratibha Chougule, 2019).

Maintaining good oral hygiene is also important for preventing tooth decay and gum disease. These conditions are caused by the build-up of plaque, a sticky film of bacteria that forms on the teeth. When plaque is not removed through regular brushing and flossing, it can lead to cavities, gum disease, and other oral health problems. By practicing good oral hygiene habits, we can prevent these conditions and maintain healthy teeth and gums. Good oral health can also have a positive impact on our mental health and well-being. People with healthy teeth and gums are more likely to feel confident and self-assured, which can improve their overall quality of life. On the other hand, people with poor oral health may feel embarrassed or ashamed, which can impact their self-esteem and social interactions (Cheng *et al.,* 2020).

Figure – 2 Causes of Oral hygiene

(https://www.who.int/newsroom/fact-sheets/detail/oral-health)

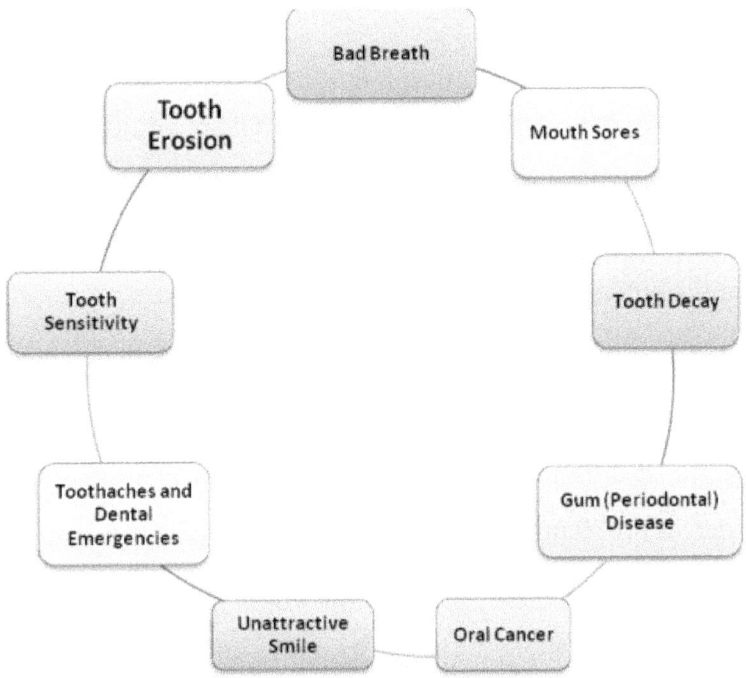

Children's dental health can have a number of detrimental implications on their physical growth, quality of life, and development (In detail Chapter -6). Oral health is particularly important for elderly people and those with impaired immune systems because they may be more susceptible to numerous oral health disorders, they should pay special attention to their oral health. The following are some ways that these populations may be impacted by oral health:

2.2.1. Enhanced Risk of Infections: People with damaged immune systems, such as the elderly, may be more prone to infections due to reduced immune systems. Untreated cavities or gum disease are examples of poor dental health that can act as a source of infection that can spread to other parts of the body.

2.2.3. Effects on Systemic Health: It is often known that good dental health contributes to general health. Diabetes and cardiovascular disease have been linked to disorders like periodontal (gum) disease, which raise the risk of these systemic illnesses. Maintaining dental health becomes even more important for immunocompromised people in order to avoid future consequences.

2.2.3. Difficulty Eating and Nutrition: Elderly and immunocompromised people may find it difficult to chew and consume a balanced diet due to oral health issues such as missing teeth, ill-fitting dentures, or mouth pain. Nutritional deficits, weight loss, and a general deterioration in health may result from this.

2.2.4. Medication-Induced dental Health Problems: Older adults and people with impaired immune systems may be administered certain drugs, which may have adverse effects on dental health. For instance, taking certain drugs may cause xerostomia, or dry mouth, which raises the risk of gum disease and cavities.

2.2.5. Chronic Conditions and Oral Health: Conditions like arthritis or cognitive impairment, which are more common in older populations, might make maintaining good oral hygiene difficult. People may find it difficult to do oral hygiene duties like brushing and flossing, which increases the risk of dental problems.

2.2.6. Reduced Salivary Flow: Certain medical disorders and aging might cause a decrease in salivary flow. Saliva is essential for preserving dental health because it helps wash away food particles, neutralize acids, and stop harmful germs from growing. A lower salivary flow can raise the risk of cavities and other oral health issues.

2.3. Factors affecting oral health

2.3.1. Eating foods that can harm your teeth: Here are a number of additional things than sugar that can harm your oral health. Given that most of us identify the following items with a healthy diet, this list may come as a surprise. It's difficult to understand that a beneficial thing could simultaneously be harmful to your dental health. Fruits with citrus peels, such as oranges, grapefruits, limes, and lemons: When ingested in excess, they can erode dental enamel. Because dried fruits are frequently sticky, they can deposit bacteria and plaque on teeth, forming a film that is difficult to remove. Similar to dried fruits, nut butters have a tendency to adhere to teeth, which can foster the growth of bacteria and plaque. The Nature of raw nuts can break teeth if you bite down on them because of how hard they are.

2.3.2. Excessive contact with certain chemicals: Regular exposure to a range of chemicals can cause dental sensitivity, discoloration, and/or damage to tooth enamel. These substances include teeth-whitening strips' ingredients, BPA (which is frequently present in canned products and plastic containers), chlorine from swimming pools, and antibiotics. Furthermore, dry mouth is a side effect of some drugs that has been linked to a higher risk of gum disease and cavities.

2.3.3. Consuming alcohol: To completely comprehend the connection between alcohol use and oral health, more research is required. Thus far, research indicates that drinking alcohol may raise the chance of developing periodontal disease, a more severe type of gum disease. Oral cancer risk may also rise as a result. Furthermore, there is a link between excessive or frequent alcohol use and poor oral hygiene, which is a significant risk factor for gum disease and cavities.

2.3.4. Chronic stress: Chronic stress has been linked to an increased risk of periodontal disease, according to studies. This could be as a result of stress producing inflammation in the body, which increases the body's susceptibility to illness, including the mouth.

2.3.5. Diabetes: Diabetes damages the blood vessels in the body. The presence of blood vessels in the gums may raise the risk of gum infections. Additionally, it may weaken the gums and increase the mouth's vulnerability to tooth loss (In detail chapter - 14).

2.3.6. Playing sports: When someone plays high-contact sports without using a mouthguard, it becomes problematic. Because teeth can be lost or damaged in collisions or other high-impact situations if they aren't adequately protected, this could jeopardize oral health. There are two ways to effectively counteract the risk factors on this list. Start by exercising moderation and balance. Secondly, make sure you regularly practice proper dental hygiene by brushing and flossing your teeth, using mouthguards when necessary, and visiting your dentist at least once every six months. The greatest method for everyone to keep their oral health is to use these tactics in tandem.

2.4. Prevention of ECC

2.4.1. Dantadhāvana literally means 'cleaning the teeth': It is one of the earliest acts in one's daily routine. It is generally done with a small piece of a twig with its bark, taken from certain specified plants or trees having medicinal properties after shaping it like a toothbrush by crushing one of its ends (Dhage and Pratibha Chougule, 2019).

2.4.2. Gandusha (gaegling) or oil pulling: Oil pulling is an ancient Ayurveda procedure that involves swishing oil in the mouth for oral and systemic health benefits. It is mentioned in the ayurvedic text Charaka Samhita where it is called kavala or gandusha.oil pulling has been used extensively as a traditional Indian folk remedy for many years to prevent decay, oral malodor, bleeding gums, dryness of throat, cracked lips and for strengthening teeth, gums and the jaw (Dhage and Pratibha Chougule, 2019).

2.4.3. Brushing: To get the best oral hygiene results from toothbrushing, use an electric toothbrush.

2.4.4. Flossing: One method that helps maintain oral hygiene b removing bacteria from areas between the teeth that are hard to reach by brushing alone is flossing. Rinsing with a mouthwash can get to place that your toothbrush and even the deep cleaning of floss can miss. Look for a mouthwash that contains fluoride, because fluoride is proven to strengthen enamel and fight cavities. In addition, a mouthwash such as crest pro-health advanced strengthens enamel, prevents cavities, and kills bad breath bacteria (Dhage and Pratibha Chougule, 2019).

2.4.5. Jivha nirlekhan (tongue scrapping): It is ideal to use gold, silver, copper, stainless steel for scrapping of the tongue. Tongue scrapping stimulates the reflex points of the tongue, removes bad color (halitosis). Improves the sense of taste, stimulate the secretion of digestive enzymes (Dhage and Pratibha Chougule, 2019).

2.4.6. General guidelines: Suggest brushing twice a day but ideally the mouth would be cleaned after every meal. Cleaning between the teeth is called interdental cleaning and is as important as tooth brushing. This is because a toothbrush cannot reach between the teeth and therefore only removes about 50% of plaque off the surface. There are many tools to clean between the teeth, including floss, flossettes, and interdental brushes (Dhage and Pratibha Chougule, 2019).

2.4.7. Diet: A nutritious, balanced diet is essential for your overall health, and it's important for your oral hygiene, too. Be sure to include plenty of dairy products, fruits, vegetables, and whole grains in your diet. Some foods that are especially good for oral hygiene: cheese, yogurt, milk, and peanuts. These foods can help remove sugars from the tooth surface and protect the teeth from plaque (Dhage and Pratibha Chougule, 2019).

References

Abhinav Singh and Bharathi Purohit. Tooth brushing, oil pulling and tissue regeneration: A review of holistic approaches to oral health. J Ayurveda Integr Med. 2011 Apr-Jun; 2(2): 64–68.

Anita M. Mark. Oral health care tips for caregivers. Volume 150, issue 5, p480, may 2019

Hina Makkar, Mark A. Reynolds, Abhishek Wadhawan, Aline Dagdag, Anwar T. Merchant, and Teodor T. Postolache. Periodontal, metabolic, and cardiovascular disease: Exploring the role of inflammation and mental health. Pteridines. 2018 Feb; 29(1): 124–163.

Karon Warren. Tooth Decay: Stages, Complications, and Treatment. Dental health. March 02, 2022.

Varsha S. Dhage and Pratibha Chougule. Importance of Oral Hygiene in Oro-Dental Diseases: A Review Study. International Journal of Research & Review (www.ijrrjournal.com). Vol.6; Issue: 12; December 2019.69-74.

Online Resources

- https://crest.com/en-us/oral-care-tips/adult/oral-hygiene-instructions-tips-products
- https://askthedentist.com/gum-disease-stages-prevention-treatment/
- https://www.who.int/news-room/fact-sheets/detail/oral-health
- https://yogacentral.in/2021/04/04/kavala-gandusha/
- https://anzmh.asn.au/blog/how-oral-problems-affect-your-self-esteem
- https://www.healthline.com/health/tooth-anatomy
- https://www.dentalhealth.org/diet-and-my-teeth
- https://www.mayoclinic.org/diseasesconditions/periodontitis/symptomscauses/syc-20354473
- https://www.news-medical.net/health/What-Are-Teeth-Made-Of.aspx
- https://www.kenhub.com/en/library/anatomy/anatomy-of-the-tooth
- https://dental.dpu.edu.in/blogs/the-surprising-benefits-of-regular-dental-check-ups

CHAPTER 3

The oral microbiota

HIGHLIGHTS

- Many different types of bacteria, including planktonic and biofilm forms, can develop in the mouth cavity.
- One type of microorganism that is present in the mouth cavity shortly after birth is lactobacilli.
- Staphylococcus species were colonized in the mouths of healthy adults; among these patients with rheumatoid arthritis, 56% showed oral carriage of *Staphylococci aureus*.
- In chronic and severe advanced dental disorders, a substantial fraction of the microbiota consisted of 17 unnamed taxa and Eubacteria sahurreum.
- *Actinomyces israelii* is the most common species isolated from humans.

The oral microbiota is a diverse population of bacteria that live in the human mouth. Bacteria, viruses, fungus, and other microorganisms are examples of microorganisms. The oral microbiota is essential for maintaining oral health, but imbalances can lead to a variety of dental and systemic health problems. The mouth cavity offers a unique and dynamic habitat for the growth of a wide range of bacteria. Many of the bacteria in the oral microbiota are helpful and help to keep the mouth healthy. Some bacteria, for example, aid in the breakdown of food particles and the promotion of digestion. Certain bacteria, by competing for resources and occupying ecological niches, also help to prevent the proliferation of hazardous germs. Oral bacteria can grow in two ways: in planktonic and biofilm forms. Only around 0.1% of oral bacteria grow in the planktonic state. Others usually aggregate and attach to the tooth surface to form an oral biofilm. The polysaccharides in the biofilm matrix are a resource that acidogenic bacteria metabolise and produce acids to initiate or progress the dental caries lesion.

Non-oral bacteria are commonly found in other parts of the human body (nares or gut). They can accidentally be introduced into the mouth by food, water, contact with animals, mouthing and chewing items, etc. Nevertheless, nowadays, there is a controversy about whether the oral cavity is an entry point or an important reservoir for this group of bacteria and whether they are merely transient or unique to this niche (Zuanazzi *et al.*, 2010; Vieira Colombo *et al.*, 2016). An imbalance of microbial flora contributes to the growth of various clinically important pathogens, that are generally considered ''non-oral'' bacteria (Al-Ahmad *et al.,* 2009; Van Winkelhoff *et al.,* 2016). Non-oral bacteria are non-resident, super-infectious microorganisms that are not generally considered a common part of the oral microbiota. Their eradication from the dental biofilms seems to be more challenging due to their higher resistance to antimicrobials, raising the probability of treatment failure and reinfection (Souto *et al.* 2006). *Enterobacteriaceae, Staphylococcus aureus, Enterococcus faecalis, Pseudomonas aeruginosa,* and *Acinetobacter baumannii* are the most extensively investigated species in the oral cavity. The existence of distinct and particular virulence factors can aid in the differentiation of these various species.

Dental caries is a chronic infection caused by normal oral microbial flora. Even though there are several types of bacteria in the oral cavity, only a certain species of bacteria can initiate dental caries and other dental infection. The bacteria which are most frequently associated with dental caries were *Streptococcus mutans*, Lactobacillus and Actinomycetes. The individual's microflora is extremely convoluted and extraordinary group of microorganisms forming various associations in the mouth thereby residing more than 700 dissimilar species (Metwalli *et al.*, 2013) Bacteria are considerably the most dominant form of microorganisms existing in the human oral cavity and few examples are *Streptococcus sanguis, Streptococcus mitis, Streptococcus mutans, Streptococcus salivarius, Lactobacillus acidophilus, Lactobacillus salivarius, Lactobacillus casei,* Staphylococcus spp, Eubacterium spp, Neisseria spp, Actinomyces spp, *Pepto-Streptococcus* spp, Micrococcus spp, etc. Among them *Streptococcus* alone forms the biggest association (In-detail chapter- 4) in the oral cavity (Bhatia and Ichhpujani, 2003).

3.1. Lactobacillus predominant microflora in Dental

Lactobacillus spp. is facultatively anaerobic, catalase-negative, Gram-positive, non-spore-forming rods that often grow better under microaerophilic conditions. Their Gram stain morphology can vary, including as short, plump rods, long, slender rods, in chains or palisades. Lactobacilli appear in the oral cavity during the first years of a child's life. Their presence depends on numerous factors such as the presence of ecological niches. Historically, lactobacilli were the first microorganisms implicated in dental caries development (Owen, 1949) They appear during the first years of a child's life, and are present in high numbers in saliva, on the dorsum of the tongue, mucous membranes, the hard palate, in dental plaque and, in fewer numbers, on tooth surfaces (Straetemans *et al.,* 1998). Lactobacilli are among the micro-organisms that can be found in the oral cavity soon after babies are born. The lactobacilli in the oral cavity of infants are believed to mainly come from the mouths of their parents, especially their mothers due to close contacts, and from the foods they eat, including milk and different fermented products. There is currently no effective means to determine the definite origin of or differentiate the types of Lactobacillus sp. In the oral cavity, lactobacilli can be found mostly in saliva, on the surface of the mucosa, the hard palate and the dorsum of the tongue. They are mostly thought to be transient in the mouth and their numbers on the tooth surfaces of healthy infants and young children are usually low (Caufield *et al.,* 2015).

Lactobacillus is not the caries initiator but plays an important role in the progression of caries. Lactobacilli tend to increase in numbers with increasing intake of fermentable sugars in the diet, a situation that is also conducive to dental caries. In individuals with active dental caries, both the diversity and prevalence of lactobacilli in dental plaque, especially the active carious sites, increase significantly, as compared to individuals who are caries-free (Badet and Thebaud, 2008). Among the Lactobacillus sp. identified from carious lesions, the most dominant species in adult and childhood dental caries, including severe early childhood caries, are *Lactobacillus casei/paracasei, Lactobacillus fermentum, Lactobacillus rhamnosus, Lactobacillus gasseri, Lactobacillus salivarius* and *Lactobacillus plantarum* (Caufield *et al.,* 2015). Most of the Lactobacillus sp. existed as cohabitants with other lactobacilli. A few species, including *Lactobacillus casei/paracasei, Lactobacillus fermentum* and *Lactobacillus salivarius,* were identified as the single occupant of the caries lesions.

3.2. Staphylococci in oral health

The oral cavity can act as a reservoir of certain pathogens that can cause systemic infections. *Staphylococcus aureus* is a gram-positive coccus that colonizes the nasal mucosa and skin of healthy individuals. Staphylococci are not generally considered to form part of the normal oral flora, and when isolated from the mouth have been viewed as transient colonisers (Marsh and Martin, 1999). Staphylococci are not believed to play a major role as intra-oral pathogens, although *Staphylococci aureus* may be involved in angular cheilitis (MacFarlane and Thelnarska, 1976). However, we have recently described a form of oral mucositis in elderly, dehydrated patients, which appears to be caused by *Staphylococci aureus* (Bagg *et al.,* 1995)). This finding has prompted a more extensive study of staphylococci in the oral flora of healthy individuals at different stages of life and in selected groups with systemic diseases which predispose to serious staphylococcal infection. Data already published revealed that 94% of healthy adults had oral colonisation with Staphylococcus spp, and 24% carried *Staphylococci aureus* in the mouth. In patients with rheumatoid arthritis, 56% demonstrated oral carriage of *Staphylococci aureus* (Jackson *et al.,* 1999). The ability of Staphylococcus spp to form a biofilm and live within certain niches allows them to develop mechanisms that increase persistence, such as the evasion of host defences and antibiotic efficacy. These microorganisms can easily be or become resistant to antibiotics and lead to superinfection.

3.3. Eubacterium species in oral infections

Most of the microorganisms that inhabit the oral cavity live in a symbiotic relationship. Symbiosis means where both the host and guest coexist mutually for the benefit of each other. Commensals of the oral cavity keep a close watch on the growth of species which may pose harm to human health. They prevent the adherence of microorganisms which can stick to the mucosa or tooth surfaces. Broadly these microorganisms belong to *Eubacteria, and* there have been a number of reports of the isolation of Eubacterium species in oral infections but because, in general, they are slow-growing and have fastidious nutritional requirements, they have not been widely studied (Wade *et al.,* 1990). *Eubacterium* is a genus of Gram-positive bacteria in the family Eubacteriaceae. These bacteria are characterised by a rigid cell wall. They may either be motile or nonmotile. Indeed, in a number of studies of the microbiota associated with periodontal disease, Eubacteriurn species are not mentioned at all while in others where they have been isolated, no attempt has been made at speciation. Nevertheless, Moore *et al* (1983) found that *Eubacteria brachy, Eubacteria nodaturn, Eubacteria timidum, Eubacteria alactolyticurn, Eubacteria sahurreum* and 17 un-named taxa made up a significant proportion of the subgingival microbiota in chronic and severe advanced periodontitis. Most of the research studies stated that Eubacterium species are subgingival microbiota and causing periodontitis. In addition, Eubacteriurn species are regularly isolated from carious dentine, endodontic infections and peri-apical infections.

3.4. Neisseria spp associated Dental inactions

Neisseria spp. are gram-negative, non-motile, and non-spore-forming bacteria belonging to the family Neisseriaceae. All members of the *Neisseria* spp., except the three subspecies of *Neisseria elongata* and *Neisseria weaveri*, occur as diplococcal bacteria with their adjacent sides flattened, resembling a kidney or coffee bean. Most species grow optimally at temperatures ranging between 35 to 37 °C, and growth is usually stimulated by carbon dioxide and humidity. Species are generally aerobic but some species may demonstrate growth under anaerobic conditions. *Neisseria* spp include both pathogenic and non-pathogenic that are found preliminary in the upper respiratory tract of humans and animals. Historically, 16S rRNA cloning experiments have found *Neisseria* species to be very abundant in the oral cavity (Aas *et al.,* 2005). Numerous commensal *Neisseria* species asymptomatically colonize oral and nasal cavity sites and are only rarely associated with disease. Shotgun metagenome sequencing has shown that commensal species have tropism for different sites in the oral cavity and oropharynx. *Neisseria subflava* is enriched on the dorsal surface of the tongue while *Neisseria mucosa* is prevalent in gingival plaque and on buccal mucosa (Donati *et al.,*2016).

3.5. Actinomyces an endogenous flora of the oral cavity

Actinomycete is a diverse category of bacteria that are gram-positive, filamentous, and grow in a branched pattern. They develop as mycelium or in large colonies. They are bacteria, yet they are a distinct category of creatures that may be examined separately. The morphological picture reveals that this bacterium is non-acid fast, anaerobic, and microphilic with filamentous branching and lives as a commensal in the human body but acts aggressively when it invades the mucosal barrier and enters the subcutaneous tissue. Actinomyces, a saprophytic component of the endogenous flora of the oral cavity, cause a suppurative, granulomatous inflammatory lesion that is locally aggressive and destructive. This infection is anatomically and clinically divided into three types; cervicofacial, pulmonary, and abdominal pelvic, with the first being the most common form. This infection is extremely unusual in the oral mucosal membranes; when present, patients exhibit classical symptoms of abscesses, sinus tract formation, and woody fibrosis. Bacteria of this genus include almost 30 species; among this *Actinomyces israelii* is the most prevalent species isolated in humans. Clinical features include its peak incidence in the fourth and fifth decades of life and male predilection with superimposition in immunocompromised individuals. Cultures and pathology are keystones of the diagnosis of this disease. Specific preventive measures along with a long-term antibiotic regime are the standard line of treatment (Rishi Thukral *et al.*, 2017).

Poor oral hygiene and periodontitis can ease the penetration of bacteria into the oral tissue. *Actinomyces* spp. are found mainly in exposed root surfaces (Rüdiger *et al.*, 2015). Due to poor oral hygiene bacterium, there were exposed to root surfaces leads to formation of actinomycotic lesions. Studies have shown coaggregations between strains of *Actinomyces viscosus* and *Actinomyces naeslundii* with oral streptococci-like *S. mitis* (McIntire *et al.*, 1978). Specific morphological arrangements in the form of corncobs have also been observed (Listgarten *et al.*,1973) which are mainly mediated by cell-surface interactions between bacterial receptors. Under physiological symbiotic conditions, these bacteria are commensals and do not cause pathologies. However, given specific dysbiotic circumstances, tissues may be damaged, invaded and opportunistic chronic or aggressive inflammatory processes may be initiated (McIntire *et al.*, 1978).

Interactions between species are required to thrive and endure in the oral cavity, where resources are limited. Some research reports revealed the physical and metabolic interactions that exist between members of the oral microbiota and non-oral species; these interactions can be mutualistic (coaggregation) to form biofilms or antagonistic to prevent the integration of a non-indigenous bacterial species. The biological mechanisms supporting these connections, however, remain unknown.

References

Aas JA, Paster BJ, Stokes LN, Olsen I, Dewhirst FE. Defining the normal bacterial flora of the oral cavity. *J Clin Microbiol.* 2005; 43:5721–32.

Alicia I Cuesta , Virginia Jewtuchowicz, María I Brusca, María L Nastri, Alcira C Rosa. Prevalence of Staphylococcus spp and Candida spp in the oral cavity and periodontal pockets of periodontal disease patients. Acta Odontol Latinoam. 2010;23(1):20-6.

Badet C, Thebaud NB. 2008. Ecology of lactobacilli in the oral cavity: a review of literature. Open Microbiol J. 2:38–48.

Bagg, M. P. Sweeney, K. Harvey Wood & A. Wiggins (1995) Possible Role of Staphylococcus aureus in Severe Oral Mucositis among Elderly Dehydrated Patients, Microbial Ecology in Health and Disease, 8:2, 51-56, DOI: 10.3109/08910609509141382.

Buket Acar, Feriha Çağlayan, Ahmet Çağkan İnkaya and Olcay Kurtulan. *Actinomyces*-associated Lesions Located in the Gingiva: Case Report of Rare Gingival Lesions. Contemp Clin Dent. 2017 Jan-Mar; 8(1): 182–184.doi: 10.4103/0976-237X.205067.

Caufield. P W , C N Schön, P Saraithong , Y Li , S Argimón. Oral Lactobacilli and Dental Caries: A Model for Niche Adaptation in Humans. J Dent Res. 2015 Sep;94(9 Suppl):110S-8S. doi: 10.1177/0022034515576052.

Donati C., Zolfo M., Albanese D., Tin Truong D., Asnicar F., Iebba V., et al. (2016). Uncovering Oral Neisseria Tropism and Persistence Using Metagenomic Sequencing. *Nat. Microbiol.* 1, 16070. doi: 10.1038/nmicrobiol.2016.70 .

Jackson SL, Vann WF, Jr, Kotch JB, Pahel BT, Lee JY. Impact of Poor Oral Health on Children's School Attendance and Performance. *Am J Public Health.* 2011; 101:1900–6.

Khalid H. Metwalli, Shariq A. Khan, Bastiaan P. Krom, and Mary Ann Jabra-Rizk. *Streptococcus mutans*, *Candida albicans*, and the Human Mouth: A Sticky Situation. PLoS Pathog. 2013 Oct; 9(10): e1003616. doi: 10.1371/journal.ppat.1003616.

Marsh, P. and Martin, M.V. (1999) The Resident Oral Microflora. In: Oral Microbiology, 4th Edition, Reed Educational and Professional Publishing Ltd., Woburn, 17-33.

Moody Kaldas, André Barghorn and Patrick R. Schmidlin. Actinomycosis as a Rare Local Manifestation of Severe Periodontitis. Case Report | Open Access. Volume 2020 | Article ID 5961452 | https://doi.org/10.1155/2020/5961452.

Moore, W. E. C., L. V. Holdeman, E. P. Cato, R. M. Smibert, J. A. Burmeister, and R. R. Ranney. 1983 Bacteriology of moderate (chronic) periodontitis in mature adult humans Infect. Immun. 42 510–515.

Nathan J. Weyand. Neisseria models of infection and persistence in the upper respiratory tract. Pathogens and Disease, 2017, Vol. 75, No. 3. 1-13.

Nawel Zaatout. Presence of non-oral bacteria in the oral cavity. Arch Microbiol. 2021; 203(6): 2747–2760. doi: 10.1007/s00203-021-02300-y.

Owen. O W. A study of bacterial counts (lactobacilli) in saliva related to orthodontic appliances; a preliminary report. Am J Orthod. 1949 Sep;35(9): 672-8.doi: 10.1016/0002-9416(49)90123-2.

Rajesh Bhatia, RL Ichhpujani. Microbiology for Dental Students. Jaypee Brothers Medical Publishers Pvt. Limited, 1 Nov 2003.

Rishi Thukral, Kirti Shrivastav, Vidhi Mathur, Animesh Barodiya, and Saurabh Shrivastav. Actinomyces: a deceptive infection of oral cavity. J Korean Assoc Oral Maxillofac Surg. 2017 Aug; 43(4): 282–285. doi: 10.5125/jkaoms.2017.43.4.282.

Sachidananda Mallya P., Shrikara Mallya. Microbiology and Clinical Implications of Dental Caries –A Review. 2020. J Evolution Med Dent Sci. ISSN - 2278-4748 / Vol. 9 / Issue 48 /. 3670-3615.

Souto. R, C.M. Silva-Boghossian, A.P. Colombo. Prevalence of *Pseudomonas aeruginosa* and Acinetobacter spp. in subgingival biofilm and saliva of subjects with chronic periodontal infection. Braz. J. Microbiol., 45 (2014), pp. 495-501

Straetemans M.M.E, C. van Loveren, J.J. de Soet, J. de Graaff and J.M. ten Cate. Colonization with Mutans Streptococci and Lactobacilli and the Caries Experience of Children after the Age of Five. J Dent Res., 1998. 77(10): 1851-1855.

Wade. W. G. (1996) The Role of Eubacterium Species in Periodontal Disease and Other Oral Infections, Microbial Ecology in Health and Disease, 9:6, 367-370, DOI: 10.3109/08910609609166480.

Zezhang T. Wen, Xiaochang Huang, Kassapa Ellepola, Sumei Liao, and Yihong Li. Lactobacilli and human dental caries: more than mechanical retention. Microbiology (Reading). 2022; 168(6): 001196. doi: 10.1099/mic.0.001196.

HIGHLIGHTS

- If there are no germs in the mouth cavity, dental caries will not develop. Among these, Streptococcal spp. is found in all human mouths at variable concentrations and can be passed from mother to kid.
- As a component of the oral flora, streptococcus mitis are commensal bacteria that inhabit the hard surfaces of the mouth cavity.
- *Streptococcus mutans* is the most common cariogenic bacterium in humans.
- *S. gordonii* is a non-pathogenic commensal streptococcus that colonizes tooth surfaces by forming dental plaque, or biofilms, in the human mouth.
- Antibiotic-resistant Viridans streptococci are becoming more and more prevalent.

CHAPTER 4

Streptococcal Dental Caries

Dental caries is a multifactorial human disease that has widely affected many populations all over the world. Dental caries will not occur if the oral cavity is free of bacteria. This is caused by accumulation of biofilm on tooth surface (Marsh *et al.*, 2006). Dental plaque is a general term for the diverse microbial community (predominantly bacteria) found on the tooth surface, embedded in a matrix of polymers of bacterial and salivary origin. These bacteria are organized into a material known as dental plaque which is yellowish coloured film on the surface of the teeth. Of the many types of bacteria in the mouth, the most caries active appear to be *Streptococcus mutans, Streptococcus mitis, Lactobacillus sp., Veillonella sp. and Actinomyces sp.* These bacteria can be transferred from mother to child and are present at varying levels in all human mouths. A variety of carbohydrates provide substrates for these organisms to grow on and the waste products of their metabolism - acids - initiate the tooth decay process by dissolving tooth enamel.

4.1. Viridians Group Streptococci

Viridians group streptococci (VGS) are inhabitants of the oral cavity, which is sterile at birth, but at the age of one year, Streptococcus species compose 70% of the cultivable oral flora and *S.salivarius*, *S.oralis* and *S.mitis* are predominant. VGS are also found in the gastrointestinal and urogential tracts. The term viridans is derived from the Latin *viridis* or green, and refer to the sheen caused by haemolysis (Alpha- Haemolysis) around the bacterial colonies on blood agar. Viridans group streptococci are divided into five major groups, which affect humans (Table 2).

Table 2 - Five major groups of Viridans group streptococci

(Jesper Hohwy *et al.*, 2001)

Streptococcus mutans group	*Streptococcus mutans, Streptococcus sorbinus, Streptococcus ratti*
Streptococcus salivarius group	*Streptococcus salivarius, Streptococcus infantarius Streptococcus vestibularis*
Streptococcous mitis group	*Streptococcus mitis Streptococcus oralis Streptococcus infantis Streptococcus cristatus Streptococcus perois*
Streptococcus sanguinis group	*Streptococcus sanguinis Streptococcus parasanguinis Streptococcus gordonii*
Streptococcus anginosus group	*Streptococcus anginosus Streptococcus intermedius Streptococcus constellatus*

4.2. Streptococcal Dental Caries

Streptococcus mutans is first described by Clark in 1924 after he isolated it from a carious lesion after that the real interest in this microbe was developed when researchers began studying dental caries in detail. Researchers have identified several hundred genes that appear to be unique to the organism. These are potential drug targets because disrupting them would disable the pathogen without harming the other bacteria in the mouth (Chetan *et al.*, 2011).

4.3. *Streptococcus mitis*

Streptococcus mitis are commensal bacteria and belongs to the viridans streptococci group that colonize hard surfaces in the oral cavity such as dental hard tissues as well as mucous membranes and are part of the oral flora. They are usually arranged in short chains in the shape of cocci (Bensing, 2001). These Gram-positive bacteria are not usually pathogenic but commonly cause bacterial endocarditis, which is the inflammation of an inner layer of the heart. *S. mitis* are alpha hemolytic, meaning it can break down red blood cells. *S. mitis* are not motile, do not form spores and lack group-specific antigens. *S. mitis* cells grow in pairs or short chains and they present an arrow-headed shape with a length of 0.5µm (Mitchell, 2011). *S. mitis* live optimally at temperatures between 30°C and 35°C, making them mesophiles. They are facultative anaerobes, which is a bacterium that makes ATP by aerobic respiration if oxygen is present but is also capable of switching to fermentation in the absence of oxygen (Kirchherr *et al.,* 2005).

The adherence and colonization by *Streptococcus mitis* can be summarized into four steps: the first two steps involve (A) the long range interaction adherence with suitable surface molecules through pili bacteria, and (B) the short range adherence of some pioneers bacteria which forms stronger bonds with the surface molecules leading to multiple adhesins. During the third step (C), the intermicrobial signalling, the formation of extracellular polymeric substance (EPS) and the nutritional adaption, give rise to a society produced by cell division and multiplication. In the last step (D) the incorporation of other microorganisms together with cell-cell signaling, intergenic coaggregation, metabolic synergy and genetic exchange, leads to the formation of a community (Nobbs *et al.*, 2009). The development of the community is dependent on many factors including adherence, signalling, nutritional adaption, and host modulation. In addition, environmental conditions such as pH, temperature, oxygen availability, organic metabolites etc. may influence *Streptococcus mitis* colonization.

4.4. *Streptococcus mutans*

S. mutans is a significant pathogen of oral cavity and initiates dental caries. This organism was isolated for the first time from the dental plaque by Clarke in 1924. The name 'mutans' was chosen because of its tendency to exhibit both coccal and rod shaped (mutant) cell morphology (Loesche, 1986). *S.mutans* belongs to the *S viridans* group, which is a poorly defined, heterologous group of the genus *Streptococcus*. Members of this group are indigenous to the oral cavity. Though the classification of this particular group is oversimplified, it includes a variety of strains with different physiological and serological characteristics comprising *S. mutans* group, *S. sanguis* group, *S. mitis* group, *S. salivarius* group and *S. milleri* group (Koneman *et al*., 1997). Many factors contribute to the cariogenicity of this organism such as rapid generation time, fermentation of wide range of carbohydrates, ability to withstand low pH, presence of enzyme glucosyl transferase that converts sucrose to glucose to enhance adhesion (Loesche, 1986).

In humans, *Streptococcus mutans* and *Streptococcus sobrinus,* are the most prevalent cariogenic bacteria (Caufield, 1997). A large number of studies support the strong association between mutans Streptococci level and the incidence of carious lesions (Tanzer, 2001). The presence of mutans Streptococci, both in dental plaque and saliva of young caries-free children, appears to be associated with an increase in caries risk (Thenisch *et al*., 2006). Early acquisition of mutans Streptococci is also a major risk factor of early childhood caries and the development of future caries (Berkowitz, 2006). *S. mutans* has been the most intensely investigated cariogenic bacterium in the literature, because of its strong correlation with dental caries and the relatively low presence without disease. This bacterium, which is considered "a specialist" in causing dental caries, possesses multiple inherent virulence properties essential for its cariogenic potential.

Acidogenicity, acid tolerance, adhesion and biofilm formation are considered the main virulence properties associated with the cariogenicity of *S. mutans* (Banas, 2004; Kuramitsu, 2001) *S. mutans* is capable of metabolizing a wide variety of sugars to lactic acids. The acids produced not only are responsible for tooth demineralization but also rapidly acidify the dental plaque environment around the bacterium. While *S. mutans* can adapt to the surrounding pH as low as pH 4.4, this vastly acidic condition is toxic to most other bacteria. The adhesion of *S. mutans* to tooth surfaces is mediated by a two-step process, involving sucrose-independent and sucrose-dependent mechanisms. Sucrose-independent adhesion to salivary pellicle is believed to initiate the attachment process, whereas sucrose-dependent adhesion may enhance bacterial colonization to the tooth surface (Banas, 2004; Kuramitsu, 2001).

Biofilm formation is an important virulence factor for *S. mutans*. The bacteria must be able to adhere to be maintained in the oral cavity (Burne, 1998). Giacaman *et al.* (2001) found there was no association between the levels of mutans streptococci in the saliva and caries status but there was an association between the amount of biofilm-forming mutans streptococci and caries incidence. When cells are growing in a biofilm bacterial susceptibility to antimicrobials is often reduced (Anderl *et al.,* 2000; Baehni and Takeuchi, 2003) and in established biofilms the antimicrobial effect is limited to the superficial layers (Zaura-Arite *et al.,* 2001). Sucrose is extremely important in *S. mutans* biofilm formation. The presence of sucrose decreases the antimicrobial susceptibility of *S. mutans,* probably due to the subsequent biofilm formation (Kreth, 2008) initially, or in the absence of sucrose, *S. mutans* adheres using ionic and lectin-like interactions. Streptococcal protein antigen P binds to salivary agglutinin glycoprotein (SAG) and SAG coated surfaces. In the presence of sucrose, glucans are synthesised by glucosyltransferases (GTFs). They form an extracellular layer of EPS that promote adhesion and biofilm formation (Banas and Vickerman, 2003).

4.5. *Streptococcus gordonii*

S. gordonii is part of the group viridians of Streptococci, non-pathogenic commensal streptococci, which are integral members of the human oral flora. These organisms colonize tooth surfaces by creating biofilms in the human mouth, also known as dental plaque. *S.gordonii* plays an integral role in initiating colonization by creating surfaces for other colonizers to adhere to. *S. gordonii* also causes bacterial endocarditis by entering the blood stream usually after oral trauma. *S. gordonii* colonizes platelet-fibrin thrombi, blood clotting agents, in damaged heart valves or endocardium leading to damage and dysfunction of the heart valves. Endocarditis can be treated with antibiotic therapy and may cause death (The Health Central Network, Inc. 2001).

Initially, *Streptococcus gordonii* initiates colonization through formation of a monospecies biofilm. The human tooth is covered by pellicle containing lipids and proteins, including salivary agglutinin glycoprotein. The receptors for salivary agglutin glycoprotein located on *S. gordonii* and other pioneer colonizers recognize and bind to the pellicle. *S. gordonii* cells, bound to the surface of the tooth, and then initiate a signal transduction pathway, known as BrfAB, which regulates adhesive activity. For current research *Streptococcus gordonii* is good candidate for a "live bacterial mucosal vaccine vector." The efficiency of *S. gordonii* in colonizing the oral cavity creates great potential for the stimulation of the mucosal immune system. *S. gordonii* can also be easily controlled genetically to produce a "fusion construct" that will enhance its stability. Another advantage is that heterologous antigens may be attached to the cell wall of *S. gordonii* thereby expressing a number of viral and bacterial antigens. Some examples of possible antigens are the E7 protein of human papillomavirus, the B subunit of *Escherichia coli* heat-labile toxin and the tetanus toxin fragment (Kotloff *et al.,* 2006).

Viridans streptococci have become increasingly resistant to antibiotics including penicillin, cephalosporin, erythromycin, and tetracycline. *S. mitis* is more resistant to antibiotics than other viridans streptococci (Wafa Achour *et al*., 2004). Viridans streptococci can transfer their resistant genes to more pathogenic pneumococci and group A streptococci. Among the viridans streptococci, *Streptococcus mitis* has been considered the species with the highest level of resistance to penicillin. Penicillin resistance in clinical isolates of *S. mitis* seems to be due to the production of altered high-molecular-mass penicillin binding proteins (PBPs) with low binding affinity for penicillin. These PBPs, encoded by chromosomal genes, are located in the cytoplasmic membrane and catalyse reactions in the final steps of bacterial peptidoglycan synthesis (Susan *et al*., 1999).

References

Dinesh. M.D, M.S. Uma, S. Meenatchisundaram, V.M. Anjali, P.S. Athira and Asitha Carmel. Streptococcal Dental Caries – A Short Review. International Journal of Current Research and Academic Review. ISSN: 2347-3215 Volume 4 Number 1 (January-2016) pp. 160-170.

Philip D Marsh· Dental plaque as a biofilm and a microbial community – implications for health and disease. BMC Oral Health. 2006; 6(Suppl 1): S14.Published online 2006 Jun 15. doi: 10.1186/1472-6831-6-S1-S14.

Sourabh Badjatia, Rini G Badjatia, K Thanveer, and Ajith CG Krishnan. Effects of Fluoride Varnish on *Streptococcus mutans* Count in Saliva. Int J Clin Pediatr Dent. 2017 Jan-Mar; 10(1): 62–66.Published online 2017 Feb 27. doi: 10.5005/jp-journals-10005-1409.

Katarina Westling. Viridans group Streptococci Septicaemia and Endocarditis. ISBN 91-7140-

Mohammed H.K.AL-Mamoori , Amer K. Hussain , Ahmed Kadem Kodeary and Ramla Abed AL-Naby. Effect of 405 nm Laser Light on the Cariogenic Bacteria Streptococcus Mutans. Journal of Babylon University/Pure and Applied Sciences/ No.(4)/ Vol.(23): 2015.187-193.

Kuramitsu H K. Virulence properties of oral bacteria: Impact of molecular biology. Current Issues in Molecular Biology 3(2):35-6. May 2001.

Ana Amoroso, Diego Demares, Marta Mollerach, Gabriel Gutkind, And Jacques Coyette. All Detectable High-Molecular-Mass Penicillin-Binding Proteins Are Modified in a High-Level ␤-Lactam-Resistant Clinical Isolate of Streptococcus mitis. Antimicrobial agents and chemotherapy, July 2001, Vol. 45, No. 7. p. 2075–2081.

Lemos JA, SR Palmer, L Zeng, ZT Wen, JK Kajfasz, IA Freires, J Abranches, and LJ Brady . The Biology of *Streptococcus mutans.* ASM Journals Microbiology SpectrumVol. 7, No. 1.

Selda Sayin Kutlu, Suzan Sacar, Nural Cevahir and Huseyin Turgut. Community-acquired Streptococcus mitis meningitis: a case report. International Journal of Infectious Diseases (2008) 12, e107—e109.

Beena Antony, Rekha.B, Anup Kumar Shetty, Thomas Kuruvilla and Ramanathan.K. Semiquantitation and characterization of streptococcus mutans from patients undergoing orthodontic treatment. J Biosci Tech, Vol 1 (2),2010, 59-63.

Robert J. Palmer, Jr. Composition and development of oral bacterial communities. Periodontol 2000. 2014 Feb; 64(1): 10.1111/j.1600-0757.2012.00453. x.

Chao Chien Chen, Lee Jene Teng, and Tsung Chain Chang. Identification of Clinically Relevant Viridans Group Streptococci by Sequence Analysis of the 16S-23S Ribosomal DNA Spacer Region. J Clin Microbiol. 2004 Jun; 42(6): 2651–2657.

David M. Krol and Kaitlin Whelan. Maintaining and Improving the Oral Health of Young Children. Pediatrics. Volume 151, number 1, January 2023: e2022060417.

Khushbu Yadav and Satyam Prakash. Dental Caries: A Microbiological Approach. Journal of Clinical Infectious Diseases & Practice. J Clin Infect Dis Pract 2:118. doi: 10.4172/2476-213X.1000118.

Hamzah Abdulrahman Salman and R. Senthikumar. Identification and Antibiogram Profile of *Streptococcus mutans* and *Streptococcus sobrinus* from Dental Caries Subjects. Journal of Applied Pharmaceutical Science 5 (06); 2015: 054-057.

Sonia Nath, Brianna Faye Poirier, Xiangqun Ju, Kostas Kapellas, Dandara Gabriela Haag, Pedro Henrique Ribeiro Santiago, and Lisa M. Jamieson. Dental Health Inequalities among Indigenous Populations: A Systematic Review and Meta-Analysis. Caries Res. 2021 Aug; 55(4): 268–287.

Mansson-Rahemtulla B, D C Baldone, K M Pruitt and F Rahemtulla. Effects of variations in pH and hypothiocyanite concentrations on S. mutans glucose metabolism. J Dent Res. 1987 Feb;66(2):486-91.

Yongwang Lin, Jiamin Chen, Xuedong Zhou and Yuqing Li . Inhibition of *Streptococcus mutans* biofilm formation by strategies targeting the metabolism of exopolysaccharides. Crit Rev Microbiol. 2021 Sep;47(5):667-677.

Marsh, P.D. 2006. Dental plaque as a biofilm and a microbial community implication for health and disease. *BMC Oral Health. 6 Suppl.* **1:** 14.

Jesper Hohwy, Jesper Reinholdt and Mogens Kilian. 2001. Population Dynamics of *Streptococcus mitis* in Its Natural Habitat. *Infection and Immunity.* **69(10)**: 6055 – 6063.

Clarke, J.K. **1924.** On the bacterial factor in the aetiology of dental caries. *Brit J Exp Pathol.* **(5):**141-147.

Mitchell, J. (2011). *Streptococcus mitis:* walking the line between commensalism and pathogenesis. *Molecular oral microbiology*, **26(2),** 89–98.

Loesche, W. J. 1986. Role of *Streptococcus mutans* in human dental decay. *Microbiol. Rev.* **50:** 353-380.

Berkowitz.R.J. Mutant Streptococci: Acquisition and transmission. *Pediartr. Dent.* 2006: **28(2):** 106-109.

Banas J. A. 2004. Virulence properties *of Streptococcus mutans*. Front. *Biosci.* **9:**1267–1277.

Susan M. Poutanen, Joyce De Azavedo, Barbara M. Willey, Donald E. Low, and Kelly S. Macdonald.. 1999. Molecular Characterization of Multidrug Resistance in *Streptococcus mitis.* Antimicrobial Agents and Chemotherapy. **43**:6. 1505-1507.

Wafa Achour, Olfa Guenni, Marguerite Fines, Roland Leclercq,and Assia Ben Hassen. 2004. *rpoB* Mutations in *Streptococcus mitis* Clinical Isolates Resistant to Rifampin. Antimicrobial Agents and Chemotherapy. **48**:(7). 2757–2759.

Zaura-Arite E. M.J, ten Cat. 2001. Confocal microscopy study of undisturbed and chlorhexidine-treated dental biofilm. *J Dent Res* **80:** 1436–1440.

CHAPTER 5

Childhood dental caries

HIGHLIGHTS

- Although the baby's mouth is completely sterile upon delivery, a number of factors related to oral hygiene affect oral hygiene and cause microorganisms to colonize the mouth cavity.
- At least five times more common than asthma, Dental caries is the most common childhood illness worldwide.
- Common oral health issues include periodontal disease, which affects 90–95% of people, and dental caries, which affects 60–80% of kids.
- The frequency of caries in children is influenced by a number of factors, including socioeconomic inequality, parental knowledge, attitudes, and behaviours, including food and hygiene habits.
- Primary, secondary, and tertiary preventative techniques must be used in conjunction with caries prevention in children, per the AAPD Guidelines.

Dental decay in young infants has most certainly existed for generations, although formal acknowledgment of the disorder known as early childhood caries only emerged in the twentieth century. Researchers and healthcare experts have noticed a rise in tooth decay among young children, particularly those from low-income families. The mid-twentieth century the increasing use of baby bottles and the introduction of sweetened baby formulae in the mid-twentieth century contributed to an increase in the prevalence of early childhood dental caries. The relationship between extended bottle-feeding, particularly at bedtime, and the development of dental caries has received attention. The current term early childhood caries (ECC) connotes a more complex disease, related to frequent sugar consumption in environment of enamel adherent bacteria that is not necessarily related to bottle feeding. Dental caries in children has been described by numerous terms and attributed depend to many aetiologies. Comforter Caries, Baby Bottle Syndrome, Nursing Bottle Caries, Nursing Caries, and Baby Bottle Tooth Decay.

Dental cavity is non communicable diseases among all age groups of Humans affecting globally and it's become most common, serious public health issue. Early child caries is defined as the presence of decayed, missing, and filled tooth surfaces in any deciduous dentition occurring in a child 71 months or younger (Baggio *et al.,* 2015). During childbirth, the baby's mouth cavity is entirely sterile, but several variables impact oral hygiene after milk feeding. Microbial, environmental, and other factors all play a role in microbial community colonization of the mouth cavity (Chapter- 2).

The factors that are currently associated with ECC are the life time of dentition oral health behaviour, feeding practices, nutritional habits status and geographic location. (Folayan *et al.,* 2015). Although dental cavity is not life-threatening, it has a deleterious impact on other diseases, and may cause dental pain, sleep disturbance, reduced weight and height development, reduced speech development, poor self-esteem or altered quality of life, and the likelihood of caries increasing in secondary dentition (Baggio *et al*., 2015).

5.1. Early child caries – Global Scenario

Worldwide, most children and an estimated 90% of adults have experienced caries, with the disease most prevalent in Latin American countries, countries in the Middle East and South Asia, and least prevalent in China. In the United States, dental caries is the most common childhood disease, being at least five times more common than asthma. It is the primary pathological cause of tooth loss in children. Between 29% to 59% of adults over the age of fifty, experience caries. The number of cases has decreased in some developed countries, and this decline is usually attributed to increasingly better oral hygiene practices and preventive measures such as fluoride treatment. Nonetheless, countries that have experienced an overall decrease in case of tooth decay continue to have a disparity in the distribution of the disease. Among children in the USA and Europe, 20% of the population endures 60% to 80% of cases of dental caries. A similarity skewed distribution of the disease id found throughout the world with some children having none or very few caries and others having a high number. Australia, Nepal and Sweden have a low incidence of cases of dental caries among children whereas cases are more numerous in Costa Rica and Slovakia (WHO, 2003 and WHO, 2009). Although the trend is not clear in developing countries, the number of dental caries has been increasing among children due to the uncontrolled intake of sugary substances, poor oral care practices, and inadequate health service utilization (Hanioka *et al.,* 2011).

5.2. Early child caries – Indian Scenario

Prevalence of dental caries is high and provision for restorative treatment is inadequate in most parts of the country. DCI's National survey is been conducted to determine the prevalence of dental diseases in different states of India. Prevalence of dental caries is 40%-80% (Very high in Northern states 85%-90%), Periodontal conditions usually increase with age and are found more in rural areas. Oral cancer and precancerous conditions are 3%-10% (Highest being in Orissa 7%). In perspective of oral health, most of the Indian populace is affected with the common oral problems like periodontal disease being 90-95% followed by dental caries affecting nearly 60%-80% of children, malocclusion about 30% and oral cancer which accounts for almost 30%-35% of the total diagnosed cancer cases. However, most of the Indian studies have shown that, greatest burden of all these oral problems is on the disadvantaged and socially marginalized people (WHO, 2011).

5.3. Etiological factors for Early child caries

Potential influence of intraoral factors, such as developmental defects of enamel, is also considered a risk factor for Early Childhood Caries The loss of surface integrity and deficiencies in mineralization may explain the higher risk of caries in children affected by developmental defects. Developmental defects are believed to be caused by some prenatal conditions and common childhood systemic illnesses. Socioeconomic factors at the community and family level, such as ethnicity and mother's schooling, are associated with Early Childhood Caries prevalence. Although the pathways by which these factors affect caries have not yet been fully clarified, it is likely that health beliefs, locus of control, and self-efficacy may at least partially explain socioeconomic disparities, as these factors exert an influence on parents' knowledge as well as their attitudes and practices, including dietary and hygiene practices undertaken with their children (Seow *et al.*, 2016).

5.4. Prevention of Early Childhood Dental

The American Academy of Pediatric Dentistry (**AAPD**) recognizes that caries-risk assessment and management proto-cols, also called care pathways, can assist clinicians with decisions regarding treatment based upon a child's age, caries risk, and patient compliance and are essential elements of con-temporary clinical care for infants, children, and adolescents. These recommendations are intended to educate healthcare providers and other interested parties on the assessment of caries risk in contemporary pediatric dentistry and aid in clinical decision-making regarding evidence- and risk-based diagnostic, fluoride, dietary, and restorative protocols.

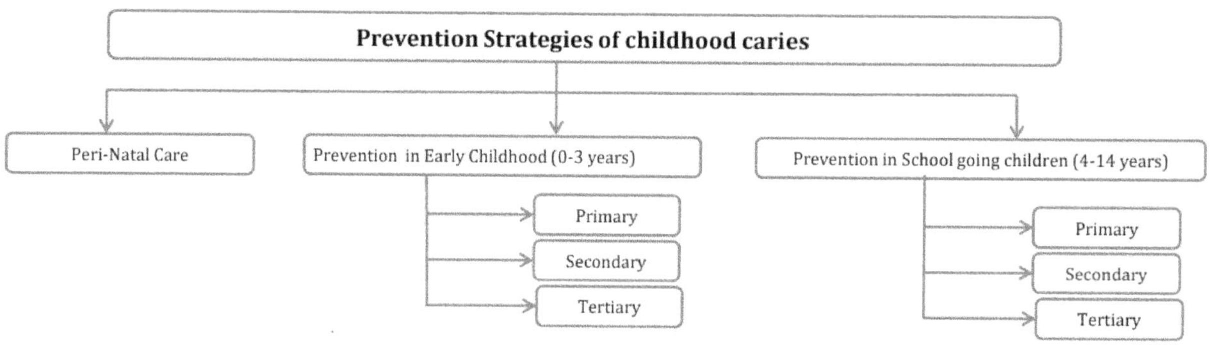

5.5. Primary prevention for ECC

Primary prevention for Early Childhood Caries needs to begin before the initiation of disease and is the key to reducing the worldwide prevalence of Early Childhood Caries. Timely delivery of educational information and preventive therapies to the parents/caregivers has been shown to be effective in reducing the prevalence of Childhood Caries.Promote primary care preventive messages that include limiting free sugar intake in foods and drink for children under 2 years; avoiding night-time bottle feeding with milk or drinks containing free sugars; and avoiding baby bottle and breastfeeding beyond 12 months, especially if frequent and/or nocturnal (Albino and Jiwari, 2016). In addition, optimal exposure to dietary fluoride is important to all dentate infants and children and can be delivered by fluoridated water, fluoridated salt, and fluoridated milk. Ideally, a child should have a dental visit for comprehensive care in the first year of life, and any child at caries risk should have regular 5% fluoride varnish applications (American Academy of Paediatric Dentistry, 2023).

5.6. Secondary prevention for ECC

Secondary prevention for ECC is preventing the progression of, or stimulating the regression (remineralization) of, caries, prior to the cavitation stage of lesions. Early detection of incipient caries is key to the prevention of cavitation. Besides the primary prevention approaches listed above, more frequent fluoride varnish applications, such as four times per year, and applying pit and fissure sealants to susceptible molars are effective non-invasive measures to arrest caries progression. Glass ionomer cements used for dental sealants have several properties favourable for use in pre-school children, such as fluoride release, chemical bonding to enamel and dentine, as well as reduced moisture sensitivity (Dhar *et al.*, 2015).

5.7. Tertiary prevention for ECC

Tertiary prevention for ECC can involve both non-invasive and invasive preventive management when there are cavitated dentine lesions. Besides all of the primary and secondary prevention approaches, silver diamine fluoride recently has gained popularity for the arrestment of cavitated lesions. The black staining of the exposed dentine due to the infiltration of silver products into the lesion, however, may limit its acceptability in certain populations. Conservative caries removal and tooth restoration may be necessary to prevent further tooth breakdown, pain, and prevent unnecessary pulp exposures (Schwendicke *et al.,* 2016). The use of atraumatic caries removal and tooth restoration with glass ionomer cement (ART) for cavitated dentine lesions is supported from studies in developing countries (American Academy of Paediatric Dentistry, 2023). The restoration of cavitated carious lesions with restorative material should be made in conjunction with the Caries Risk Assessment free materials bond to tooth structure and release fluoride which inhibits secondary caries (Dhar *et al.*, 2015).

References

Albino. J· T Tiwari, Preventing Childhood Caries: A Review of Recent Behavioural Research. J Dent Res. 2016 Jan;95(1):35-42. doi: 10.1177/0022034515609034.

American Academy of Paediatric Dentistry. Guideline on Caries-risk Assessment and Management for Infants, Children, and Adolescents. 2014. Reference Manual. V 38 / NO 6 16 / 17.

Clinical Affairs Committee – Infant Oral Health Subcommittee. Guideline on Infant Oral Health Care. Revised 2012.

Donat Uwayezu, Agnes Gatarayiha, and Manassé Nzayirambaho. Prevalence of dental caries and associated risk factors in children living with disabilities in Rwanda: a cross sectional study. Pan Afr Med J. 2020; 36: 193.doi: 10.11604/pamj.2020.36.193.24166.

Khushbu Yadav and Satyam Prakash. Dental Caries: A Review. Asian Journal of Biomedical and Pharmaceutical Sciences, 6(53), 2016, 01-07.

Lee Seng Esmond Seow n, Janhavi Ajit Vaingankar, Edimansyah Abdin, Rajeswari Sambasivam, Anitha Jeyagurunathan, Shirlene Pang, Siow Ann Chong, Mythily Subramaniam. Positive mental health in outpatients with affective disorders: Associations with life satisfaction and general functioning. Journal of Affective Disorders 190 (2016) 499–507.

Morenike O Folayan, Kikelomo A Kolawole, Elizabeth O Oziegbe, Titus Oyedele, Olusegun V Oshomoji, Nneka M Chukwumah, and Nneka Onyejaka. Prevalence, and early childhood caries risk indicators in preschool children in suburban Nigeria. BMC Oral Health. 2015; 15: 72. doi: 10.1186/s12903-015-0058-y.

Niha Dhar, Sumeer Razdan, Satiander Rana, Wajid W. Bhat, Ram Vishwakarma, and Surrinder K. Lattoo. A Decade of Molecular Understanding of Withanolide Biosynthesis and *In vitro* Studies in *Withania somnifera* (L.) Dunal: Prospects and Perspectives for Pathway Engineering. Front Plant Sci. 2015; 6: 1031. doi: 10.3389/fpls.2015.01031.

Ramya z, KVV Prasad, Niveditha H. Public oral primary preventive measures: An Indian perspective. J. Int Oral Health. 2011. Volume 3; Issue 5:1-12.

Schwendicke F, J E Frencken, L Bjørndal, M Maltz, D J Manton, D Ricketts, K Van Landuyt, A Banerjee, G Campus, S Doméjean, M Fontana, S Leal, E Lo, V Machiulskiene, A Schulte, C Splieth, A F Zandona and N P T Innes. Managing Carious Lesions: Consensus Recommendations on Carious Tissue Removal. Adv Dent Res. 2016 May;28(2):58-67. doi: 10.1177/0022034516639271.

Stéphanie Baggio, Katia Iglesias, Stéphane Deline, Joseph Studer, Yves Henchoz, Meichun Mohler-Kuo, Gerhard Gmel. Not in Education, Employment, or Training status among young Swiss men. Longitudinal associations with mental health and substance use. J Adolesc Health. 2015 Feb;56(2):238-43. doi: 10.1016/j.jadohealth.2014.09.006.

Takashi Hanioka, Miki Ojima, Keiko Tanaka, Mito Yamamoto. Does second hand smoke affect the development of dental caries in children? A systematic review. Int J Environ Res Public Health. 2011 May;8(5):1503-19. doi: 10.3390/ijerph8051503.

Taufan Bramantoro, R. Darmawan Setijanto, Retno Palupi, Achmad Zamzam Aghazy, and Wahyuning Ratih Irmalia. Dental Caries and Associated Factors among Primary School Children in Metropolitan City with the Largest Javanese Race Population: A Crosssectional Study. Contemp Clin Dent. 2019 Apr-Jun; 10(2): 274–283. doi: 10.4103/ccd.ccd_517_18.

Zi En Lim, Henry F. Duncan, Advan Moorthy and David McReynolds. Minimally invasive selective caries removal: a clinical guide. (2023). *British Dental Journal* volume 234, pages233–240.

Online Resources

https://flipper.diff.org/app/items/info/472

https://iapdworld.org/wp-content/uploads/2020/02/Tinanoff_et_...

https://iapdworld.org/wp-content/uploads/2020/04/02_Manage...

CHAPTER 6

Aetiology of Dental Caries

HIGHLIGHTS

- The main variables promoting the development of caries are plaque-producing bacteria, the natural vulnerability of tooth surfaces, eating frequency, snacking habits, dental hygiene habits, fluoride availability, and salivary flow and composition.
- A diet high in sugar speeds up the growth of several oral bacteria and alters the microflora's makeup in a way that promotes dental cavities.
- By successfully preventing thousands of tooth extractions, the installation of a sugar tax has been revealed by researchers as a substantial advancement in oral health.
- Nicotine exposure and cigarette smoking encourage the growth of caries-prone environments and the cariogenic activity of oral bacteria.

Many factors influence caries development, including the presence of plaque-producing bacteria, innate susceptibility of tooth surfaces, frequency of eating, snacking behaviour, oral hygiene practices, fluoride availability, and salivary flow and composition. All carbohydrates, including starchy foods, especially highly processed starches in savoury snacks, and foods containing sugars such as cakes, biscuits, jam, honey, fruits and fruit juices can be used by bacteria to produce acids, which accelerate demineralisation of tooth enamel. Saliva contains protective minerals (calcium and phosphates) that buffer the bacterial acids and promote remineralisation. The greater the salivary flow, the more rapid the remineralisation. It is the balance between acid production and salivary recovery that determines susceptibility to caries.

6.1. Diet and Dental caries

Diet also plays a significant aetiological role in dental erosion, the prevalence of which seems to be increasing, and dietary components may contribute to development of enamel defects (e.g. enamel hypoplasia, fluorosis). According to Sheiham (2001), "sugars, particularly sucrose, are the most important dietary aetiological cause of caries and the main strategy to further reduce the levels of caries is reducing the frequency of sugars intakes in the diet". A sucrose-rich diet increases the growth rate of many oral bacteria and changes the composition of the microflora in a caries-promoting manner (Marsh and Nyvad, 2001). Repeated acid attacks which do not give teeth the time to recover increase risk of caries, so small amounts of sugar and other fermentable carbohydrates eaten frequently during the day will increase caries risk more than large amounts eaten infrequently. Additionally, the amount of sugar consumed is less important than how quickly it is cleared from the mouth. Sticky foods like breads or raisins stay in the mouth much longer, and increase the potential for decay. Calcium rich foods like cheese, eaten immediately after sugar, can help protect against demineralisation. The relationship between the amount of sugar consumed and the levels of decay in individuals is actually very weak.

6.2. Consumption of dietary carbohydrates

Consumption of dietary carbohydrates is one of the most important etiological factors as they are processed by bacteria in the dental plaque via the glycolytic pathway producing acids, mainly lactate (Konig and Navia, 1995). Frequent and prolonged exposure of the teeth to dietary carbohydrates generates an acidic plaque environment, which promotes the demineralization of the dental enamel, causing caries. In addition, frequent consumption of simple carbohydrates promotes the overgrowth of cariogenic bacteria in the dental plaque, such as the mutans streptococci and the lactobacilli, as these are more resistant to acidic environments than the less cariogenic species [Marsh, 1991]. This explains how diets rich in sugars increase the risk of caries [Campain *et al.*, 2003]. In fact, the World Health Organization in 2015 published a guideline on sugar intake, recommending an intake of free sugars (includes added sugars as well as sugars naturally present in fruit juices as well as fruit juice concentrates) below 10% of total energy intake [WHO, 2015]. This recommendation was based on an analysis of cohort studies in children showing higher rates of dental caries with greater than 10% of total energy intake from free sugars compared to less than 10%.

The cariogenic potential of a carbohydrate depends mainly on how efficiently it can be metabolised by oral bacteria through the glycolytic pathway, which is reflected by the intensity of acidification that it induces in dental plaque [Maehara *et al.*, 2005]. For example, monosaccharides such as glucose and fructose can enter the glycolytic pathway directly after being converted to fructose-1,6-biphosphate, while more complex carbohydrates such as starch, first need to be broken down into more simple sugars before entering glycolysis. Consequently, glucose and fructose induce a faster and more pronounced pH drop in the dental plaque than starch, and are more cariogenic [Bibby and Krobicka, 1984]. The milk sugar lactose produces a smaller pH drop in plaque compared to glucose, fructose, and sucrose; consequently, milk is less cariogenic [Johansson and Lif Holgerson, 2011]. Table sugar (sucrose) is considered the most cariogenic sugar, not only because it usually produces the most pronounced pH drop in plaque, but also because it can serve as a substrate for the synthesis of extracellular (EPS) and intracellular (IPS) polysaccharides by oral bacteria [Lingstrom *et al.*, 2000; Newbrun, 1967; Bowen, 2002]. The insoluble glucans can facilitate bacterial adherence [Schilling and Bowen, 1992] and can increase the porosity of the plaque, which allows sugar and bacteria to diffuse deep along the tooth structure [Shellis and Dibdin, 1988], forming a "sticky" plaque compared to the plaque formed in the absence of sucrose.

Researchers unveil a significant breakthrough in oral health as implementation of a sugar tax has successfully prevented thousands of tooth extractions. A positive outcome reflects the tangible impact of policy measures aimed at curbing excessive sugar consumption as a new study has highlighted how the UK Soft Drinks Industry Levy or the taxation introduced in 2018 of sugary products, has not only contributed to improved public health but has also served as a preventive measure, reducing the need for invasive dental procedures. The tax required the manufacturers of drinks with over 5g of sugar to pay a 'sugar tax' and now, a findings from a new research published in BMJ Nutrition, Prevention & Health underscores the effectiveness of public health initiatives in addressing the oral health challenges associated with high sugar intake, marking a noteworthy stride in promoting overall well-being (Zarafshan Shiraz, New Delhi - Nov 15, 2023)

The World Health Organization tagged dental caries (also known as tooth decay or dental cavities) as the most common noncommunicable disease worldwide that affects general health and often causes pain and infection, which may result in tooth extraction while its severity is a frequent cause of absenteeism at school or work. The WHO stated that in many countries, sugars-sweetened beverages, including fruit-based and milk-based sweetened drinks and 100% fruit juices, are a primary source of free sugars, as well as confectionery, cakes, biscuits, sweetened cereals, sweet desserts, sucrose, honey, syrups and preserves but limiting free sugars intake to less than 10% of total energy intake – and ideally even further, to less than 5% –

minimises the risk of dental caries throughout the life course (Zarafshan Shiraz, New Delhi - Nov 15, 2023)

To inform the process of the Global Strategy on Oral health where the WHO is exploring cost-effective interventions for oral health, including taxation on sugar-sweetened beverages (SSBs), an umbrella review was conducted. The team looked at data from 2012, before the tax was introduced, to February 2020 and it was found that the number of under 18s having a tooth removed due to decay may have fallen by 12% as a result. Based on a population of nearly 13 million children in England in 2020, the researchers estimated that the reduction avoided 5,638 admissions for tooth decay while the reductions in hospital admissions were greatest in younger children aged up to four years and among children aged five to nine years, with absolute reductions of 6.5 and 3.3 per 100,000 respectively. Study's first by Nina Rogers from MRC Epidemiology Unit at the University of Cambridge, said that, "This is an important finding given that children aged five to nine are the most likely to be admitted to hospital for tooth extractions under general anaesthesia" (Zarafshan Shiraz, New Delhi - Nov 15, 2023)

6.3. Correlation between tobacco Smoking and Dental caries

Tobacco is detrimental to human health. The latest Surgeon General's Report (SGR), 'The Health Consequences of Smoking–50 Years of Progress', updated the evidence of the infaust effects of smoking on health (Centers for Disease Control and Prevention, 2014). The World Health Organization (WHO) estimates that tobacco is responsible for more than 7 million deaths and hundreds of billions of dollars loss, worldwide each year (*WHO, 2017)*. More than 60 toxic chemicals in tobacco such as nicotine can invade the body's multiple systems (Mitali *et al.,* 2016). They lead to cardiovascular diseases, cancers and other systemic diseases (Selwitz *et al.,* 2017). In addition, tobacco is a harmful product responsible for adverse oral conditions and some oral diseases. Any form of tobacco consumption is responsible for oral diseases like adult periodontal diseases, oral cancer, cleft lip, cleft palate and other congenital defects in children whose mothers smoked tobacco during pregnancy (Petersen , 2003). An increasing number of studies have focused on the association between tobacco smoking and dental caries.

Numerous epidemiological studies around the world have reported a close relationship between smoking and the occurrence of dental caries. In Italy, smoking military personnel (including 94.6% men and 5.4% women) have a higher decayed, missing, filled teeth (DMFT) score than non-smoking personnel (Campus *et al.,* 2015). In Finland, daily smoking has been found to increase 4-year caries experience in adults (Bernabé *et al.*, 2015). A study in Scotland has shown that if a pregnant woman smokes it might result in her child having a higher prevalence of caries than a child born to a non-smoking mother (Bernabé *et al.,* 2017). In Portugal, smoking has been confirmed as a risk factor for dental caries, and avoiding exposure to smoking leads to a 7% decrease in caries incidence[4]. A systematic review by Benedetti et al (Benedetti *et al.*, 2013). also verified that tobacco smoking had a close association with an increased risk of caries. However, there were differences between smokers and non-smokers in regard to personal education and economic situation[6]. Investigation showed that smokers tended to have bad eating habits, payed less attention to oral self-care, rarely seeking professional medical treatment and had poor compliance after treatment. All these behaviours mentioned above could increase the incidence of caries (Axelsson *et al.,* 1998). Cigarette smoking and nicotine exposure promote the cariogenic activity of oral microorganisms and the formation of a caries-susceptible environment. This suggests that smokers should quit smoking, amongst other health reasons, also for their oral health.

References

Axelsson P, Paulander J, Lindhe J. Relationship between smoking and dental status in 35-, 50-, 65-, and 75-year-old individuals. J Clin Periodontol. 1998 Apr;25(4):297-305.

Efka Zabokova Bilbilova. Dietary Factors, Salivary Parameters, and Dental Caries. DOI: 10.5772/intechopen.92392

Fabrizio Benedetti. Placebo and the New Physiology of the Doctor-Patient Relationship. Physiol Rev93: 1207–1246, 2013.

Jiang X, Jiang X, Wang Y, Huang R. Correlation between tobacco smoking and dental caries: A systematic review and meta-analysis. Tob Induc Dis. 2019 Apr 19; 17:34.

Kassebaum NJ, Bernabé E, Dahiya M, Bhandari B, Murray CJL, Marcenes W. Global Burden of Untreated Caries: A Systematic Review and Metaregression. *Journal of Dental Research.* 2015;94(5):650-658.

Kivela J, Parkkila S, Parkkila AK, Leinonen J, Rajaniemi H. Salivary carbonic anhydrase isoenzyme VI. J Physiol. 1999 Oct 15;520 Pt 2(Pt 2):315-20.

König KG, Navia JM. Nutritional role of sugars in oral health. Am J Clin Nutr. 1995 Jul;62(1 Suppl):275S-282S; discussion 282S-283S.

Lemos JA, Palmer SR, Zeng L, Wen ZT, Kajfasz JK, Freires IA, Abranches J, Brady LJ. The Biology of *Streptococcus mutans*. Microbiol Spectr. 2019 Jan;7(1):10.1128/ microbiolspec. GPP3-0051-2018.

Lif Holgerson P, Harnevik L, Hernell O, Tanner AC, Johansson I. Mode of birth delivery affects oral microbiota in infants. J Dent Res. 2011 Oct;90(10):1183-8.

Lenander-Lumikari and V. Loimaranta. Saliva and Dental Caries. Adv Dent Res 14:40-47, December, 2000

Marsh PD. Dental plaque as a biofilm and a microbial community - implications for health and disease. BMC Oral Health. 2006 Jun 15;6 Suppl 1(Suppl 1): S14.

Marsh PD. Are dental diseases examples of ecological catastrophes? *Microbiology.* 2003; 149:279–294.

Palacios C, Rivas-Tumanyan S, Morou-Bermúdez E, Colon AM, Torres RY, Elías-Boneta AR. Association between Type, Amount, and Pattern of Carbohydrate Consumption with Dental Caries in 12-Year-Olds in Puerto Rico. Caries Res. 2016;50(6):560-570.

Paula Moynihan, and Poul Erik Petersen. Diet, nutrition and the prevention of dental diseases. Public Health Nutrition: 7(1A), 201–226.

Petersen PE. The World Oral Health Report 2003: continuous improvement of oral health in the 21st century--the approach of the WHO Global Oral Health Programme. Community Dent Oral Epidemiol. 2003 Dec;31 Suppl 1:3-23.

Roberto Pinna, Guglielmo Campus, Enzo Cumbo, Ida Mura & Egle Milia (2015) Xerostomia induced by radiotherapy: an overview of the physiopathology, clinical evidence, and management of the oral damage, Therapeutics and Clinical Risk Management, 11: 171-188

Sheiham. A. Dietary effects on dental diseases. Public Health Nutri. 2001 Apr;4(2B):569-91. doi: 10.1079/phn2001142.

Shellis RP, Dibdin GH. Analysis of the buffering systems in dental plaque. J Dent Res. 1988 Feb;67(2):438-46.

Shigetada Kawabata and Shigeyuki Hamada. [37] Studying biofilm formation of mutanss streptococci. Methods in Enzymology Volume 310, 1999, Pages 513-523

Stuart G. Dashper and Eric C Reynolds. Effects of Organic Acid Anions on Growth, Glycolysis, and Intracellular pH of Oral Streptococci. February 2000 Journal of Dental Research 79(1):90-6

Tomonori Hoshino and Taku Fujiwara. The findings of glucosyltransferase enzymes derived from oral streptococci. japanese Dental Science Review 58 (2022) 328–335.

Warren GW, Alberg AJ, Kraft AS, Cummings KM. The 2014 Surgeon General's report: "The health consequences of smoking--50 years of progress": a paradigm shift in cancer care. Cancer.

Wu J, Li M, Huang R. The effect of smoking on caries-related microorganisms. Tob Induc Dis. 2019 Apr 18; 17:32.

CHAPTER 7

Sign and Symptoms

HIGHLIGHTS

- In certain instances, particularly when dental decay advances slowly, there may be no pain at all.
- Sensitivity to cold foods is a marker of dental cavities, but it also shows that the tooth is still alive.
- Teeth that have darkened are indicative of dental decay because the dying or dead pulp releases specific pigments that give the teeth their dark appearance.
- When a tooth becomes decayed Applying pressure could cause discomfort and anguish. Upper back tooth discomfort can occasionally be caused by sinus infections.
- Cavities can make bad breath worse. Cavity formation is usually associated with oral bacteria.

A person experiencing caries may not be aware of the disease. Pain due to dental caries can range from mild to severe depending on its progress. In some cases, if the decay progresses very slowly, pain may be totally absent too. The earliest sign of a new carious lesion is the appearance of a chalky white spot on the surface of the tooth, indicating an area of demineralization of enamel. This is referred to as incipient decay. As the lesion continues to dematerialize, it can turn brown but will eventually turn into a cavitations ("cavity"). Before the cavity forms, the process is reversible, but once a cavity forms, the lost tooth structure cannot be regenerated. A lesion that appears brown and shiny suggests dental caries were once present but the demineralization process has stopped, leaving a stain. A brown spot that is dull in appearance is probably a sign of active caries.

One of the signs of dental cavities, sensitivity to cold foods is an indication that the tooth is still alive. There is a possibility of saving the tooth with a filling if treated on time. However, if feel sensitivity and pain when consume anything hot, it may be a sign of a dying or dead tooth. Teeth chipping off when bite or chew on anything moderately hard; it may be a sign of dental decay. The way the enamel (outermost layer of the tooth) and dentine (the second layer of the tooth) are structured, when the decay progressed to dentin, it undermines the overlying enamel. This makes the enamel vulnerable to fractures. **Darkening of teeth** is a sign of dental decay. Basically, when the decay progresses to the pulp, there is a lot of destruction of the dentine. This coupled with the fact that the dying or dead pulp produces certain pigments makes the teeth look dark. When the dental decay reaches the pulp of the tooth and then progresses to the tissues surrounding it along with the bone, it generates pus. This can cause swelling in the gums and often has to be treated immediately. As the enamel and dentin are destroyed, the cavity becomes more noticeable. The affected areas of the tooth change color and become soft to the touch. Once the decay passes through enamel, the dentinal tubule, which have passages to the nerve of the tooth become exposed and causes a tooth ache. The pain may worsen with exposure to heat, cold, or sweet foods and drinks. Dental caries can also cause bad breath and foul tastes. In highly progressed cases, infection can spread from the tooth to the surrounding soft tissues. Complications such as cavernous sinus_thrombosis and Ludwig's angina can be life-threatening. Some common sign and symptoms are described below.

7.1. Tooth sensitivity

One dental condition that is frequently experienced by many people is tooth sensitivity. It happens when the layer of enamel covering your teeth thins or when gum recession reveals the dentin, which is the underlying surface. Little tubules in the dentin connect to the nerve core of the tooth. When these tubules are exposed, pain or discomfort may result, particularly when certain triggers are applied. Using a hard-bristled toothbrush or applying excessive force when brushing your teeth will gradually wear down the enamel, exposing the dentin. Over time, eating and drinking acidic foods and drinks can erode enamel and cause sensitivity. A transient sensitivity may be experienced after certain dental procedures, such as teeth whitening or tooth replacement. When teeth crack, the dentin may be exposed, which can cause sensitivity. Cavities have the potential to reveal the teeth's delicate inner layers.

7.2. Tooth pain when eating or drinking

Tooth pain during eating or drinking can result from a number of dental problems. Finding the underlying reason of this kind of discomfort is crucial if you're feeling it. The following are a few possible causes of tooth pain during eating or drinking: Cavities are dental decay places that might hurt, particularly when you consume hot, cold, or sweet foods or beverages. Eating can be painful for a tooth that has cracked or fractured because of its sensitivity to pressure or temperature changes. Foods and drinks that are hot, cold, sweet, or acidic can cause sensitivity in exposed dentin, which is frequently the result of gum recession or enamel erosion. An infection at a tooth's root is called an abscess. Particularly when chewing or ingesting hot or cold things, it can produce excruciating agony. Gum recession brought on by advanced gum disease (periodontitis) can reveal the tooth roots and cause discomfort when eating or drinking. Chewing may be painful crowns, dental fillings, or other restorations that are ill-fitting or broken. Pain and discomfort, particularly when eating or drinking, can be caused by impacted wisdom teeth. An upper back toothache may occasionally be connected to a sinus infection.

7.3. Tooth pain when pressure

Pressure-induced tooth pain is frequently an indication of a more serious dental problem. This kind of discomfort can be brought on by a number of conditions, so it's critical to pinpoint the exact source in order to receive the right care. Cavities are patches of dental enamel deterioration. Pressure can be painful or uncomfortable when it is applied, like while chewing. A tooth that has cracked or broken may be pressure-sensitive. Biting down on food may make the pain more apparent. A bacterial infection near the tooth's root causes an abscess. It can hurt a lot, especially when pressure is applied. An unpleasant taste in the mouth and puffiness are possible additional symptoms. Pockets between the gums and teeth may develop as a result of advanced gum disease. Applying pressure might result in pain and discomfort. When wisdom teeth or other teeth erupt, pressure can cause pain during the eruption process. When pressure is applied, sinus infections can occasionally result in pain in the upper back teeth. We call this transferred pain. When chewing, pressure points on the temporomandibular joint, which joins the jaw to the skull, may become painful.

7.4. Discoloration or Stain on Teeth

Teeth discoloration or staining can result from a variety of causes, and the right course of action depends on the particular reason. Surface stains on teeth can be caused by external causes such as food, drinks (coffee, tea, red wine), tobacco, and inadequate dental hygiene. Consistent brushing, flossing, and expert dental cleanings can assist in eliminating these external stains. Internal factors such as aging, trauma, some drugs, or excessive fluoride during tooth formation. Gray or brown discolouration may arise from the use of tetracycline antibiotics throughout the period of teeth development in children. Tooth discolouration or black patches can be brought on by cavities and tooth decay. Over time, teeth that have received root canal therapy may seem darker. Genetic factors may cause some people to naturally have teeth that are darker or more yellow in colour.

7.5. Cavities Lead to Bad Breath

Bad breath can be exacerbated by cavities. Bacteria in the mouth are frequently linked to the formation of cavities. Cavities or dental caries may develop as a result of bacteria breaking down food particles and producing acids. Bad breath can be caused by an offensive stench that is produced by bacteria in and around cavities as well as food particles that are decomposing. Furthermore, the development of an abscess may result from a cavity that worsens and infects the pulp, which is the tooth's inner layer. An abscess is a pocket of pus that can cause poor breath and release an unpleasant odour.

Online Resources

- https://www.thehealthsite.com/oral-health/signs-of-dental-cavities-68448/
- https://bio.libretexts.org/Bookshelves/Microbiology/Microbiology_(Boundless)/15:_Diseases/15.07:_Bacterial_Diseases_of_the_Mouth/15.7B:_Dental_Caries
- https://www.listerine.com/cavities-strong-teeth/7-signs-cavities
- https://my.clevelandclinic.org/health/symptoms/10954-teeth-sensitivity
- https://ada.com/conditions/dental-abscess/
- https://www.mayoclinic.org/diseases-conditions/acute-sinusitis/expertanswers/toothache/faq-20058299
- https://www.dentalhealth.org/sensitive-teeth
- https://www.ida.org.in/Public/Details/Brushing

CHAPTER 8

Epidemiology

HIGHLIGHTS

- From an epidemiological perspective, dental caries is a global issue that may be classified as a public health emergency.
- From the standpoint of dental health, 90%–95% of Indians suffer from common oral conditions such caries disease.
- In certain developed nations, the number of cases has declined, and this decrease is typically attributable to improved preventative and oral hygiene practices.
- Dental caries can be avoided by taking easy steps and raising public knowledge of them in a timely manner.
- Data on the prevalence of dental caries in Indian populations across various age groups, geographic regions, dentitions, and diagnostic criteria are generally needed.

From an epidemiological point of view, dental caries is widely disseminated across the world and may be considered a public health problem in world wide. Dental diseases are one of the most common of non-communicable diseases. Though they are rarely life threatening, they do impact the quality of life. Thus, they are an important public health concern. According to the World Health Organization (WHO), the prevalent oral diseases are dental caries, periodontal diseases and edentulousness.

Prevalence of dental caries is high and provision for restorative treatment is inadequate in most parts of the country. DCI's National survey is been conducted to determine the prevalence of dental diseases in different states of India. Prevalence of dental caries is 40%-80% (Very high in Northern states 85%-90%), Periodontal conditions usually increase with age and are found more in rural areas. Oral cancer and precancerous conditions are 3%-10% (Highest being in Orissa 7%). In perspective of oral health, most of the Indian populace is affected with the common oral problems like periodontal disease being 90-95% followed by dental caries affecting nearly 60%-80% of children, malocclusion about 30% and oral cancer which accounts for almost 30%-35% of the total diagnosed cancer cases. However, most of the Indian studies have shown that, greatest burden of all these oral problems is on the disadvantaged and socially marginalized people (WHO, 2011). Dental caries is still one of the most common diseases in the world today. Until recently almost everyone had experienced tooth decay in their lifetime. However, today many people are caries free and there has been a 40%-60 % reduction in the incidence of tooth decay around the Western world. Most developed countries and many non-industrialized countries are now well below the World Health Organization goal of less than 3 decayed, missing or filled teeth per 12-year-old child (WHO, 2003).

Worldwide, most children and an estimated 90% of adults have experienced caries, with the disease most prevalent in Latin American countries, countries in the Middle East and South Asia, and least prevalent in China. In the United States, dental caries is the most common childhood disease, being at least five times more common than asthma. It is the primary pathological cause of tooth loss in children. Between 29% to 59% of adults over the age of fifty, experience caries. The number of cases has decreased in some developed countries, and this decline is usually attributed to increasingly better oral hygiene practices and preventive measures such as fluoride treatment. Nonetheless, countries that have experienced an overall decrease in case of tooth decay continue to have a disparity in the distribution of the disease. Among children in the USA and Europe, 20% of the population endures 60% to 80% of cases of dental caries. A similarity skewed distribution of the disease found throughout the world with some children having none or very few caries and others having a high number. Australia, Nepal and Sweden have a low incidence of cases of dental caries among children whereas cases are more numerous in Costa Rica and Slovakia (WHO, 2003 and WHO, 2009).

In the year 2016, the first attempt was made to assess the state-wise global disease burden (GDB) of India. The results of this study showed that the five leading individual causes of disability-adjusted life years (DALYs) in India were ischemic heart disease, chronic obstructive pulmonary disease, diarrheal diseases, lower respiratory infections, and cerebrovascular disease (Dandona *et al*., 2017). Oral health was totally overlooked and not recorded in this survey. Many oral diseases like oral cancers, periodontal diseases, and dental caries have high prevalence in India and are a matter of concern. There are many factors that these include (Chapter- 6) not only these but low socioeconomic status, less education, unavailability of dental insurance coverage, and prolonged orthodontic treatment especially with fixed braces and poorly fabricated partial dentures have also been associated with dental caries in Inda. Dental caries is one of the leading causative agents of oral agony and the prime reason for patients to visit dental clinics or hospitals. Unfortunately, the patients report at a stage when some amount of loss of the tooth structure has already taken place. In early stages, restorations can be done to save the tooth, but in later stages, root canal treatment or extractions are the only resorts. People are susceptible to dental caries throughout their lives.

The scenario in India is no different from other developed or developing countries (Alsuraim and Han, 2020). The dentist population ratio in India ranges from 1:1000 to 1:20,000 across different states (Padminee *et al.*, 2020). Annually, 30,570 dentists are produced in India; however, only 10% of dentists serve the rural people (Chandu *et al.,* 2017). With a poor dentist to population ratios in some areas, the chances of dental caries going undiagnosed are highly likely, contributing the regional disparity in dental caries prevalence rates (Parasuraman *et al.,* 2017). Hence a true prevalence rate needs to be elucidated in order to address the growing concern of dental caries. Generally, there was no data on the pooled prevalence of dental caries among Indian population from different age groups, geographical region, dentition, and diagnostic criteria.

References

Bakr Salem Alsuraim and Dong-Hun Han. Effect of globalization on global dental caries trend. Medicine (Baltimore). 2020 Aug 28; 99(35): e21767.doi: 10.1097/MD.0000000000021767.

Batra P, Saini P and Yadav V. Oral health concerns in India. J Oral Biol Craniofac Res. 2020 Apr-Jun;10(2):171-174.

Chan AKY, Tamrakar M, Jiang CM, Lo ECM, Leung KCM, Chu CH. A Systematic Review on Caries Status of Older Adults. Int J Environ Res Public Health. 2021 Oct 12;18(20):10662.

Chandu VC, Pachava S, Viswanath V. Strategies for improving accessibility to oral health care services in rural India: An insight. *Int J Oral Health Med Res.* 2017; 4:44–6.

Dandona R, Bertozzi-Villa A, Kumar GA, Dandona L. Lessons from a decade of suicide surveillance in India: who, why and how? Int J Epidemiol 2017; 46: 983–93.

Krishnan Padminee, R. Anusha, Krishnan Lakshmi, Parangimalai Diwakar Madan Kumar. Geographic disproportions in dental workforce distribution and its impact on oral disease burden: An Indian perspective. SRM Journal of Research in Dental Sciences. 2020, IP: 157.46.34.96.

Miglani S. Burden of Dental Caries in India: Current Scenario and Future Strategies. Int J Clin Pediatr Dent. 2020 Mar-Apr;13(2):155-159.

Pandey P, Nandkeoliar T, Tikku AP, Singh D and Singh MK. Prevalence of Dental Caries in the Indian Population: A Systematic Review and Meta-analysis. J Int Soc Prev Community Dent. 2021 Jun 10;11(3):256-265.

Ramya K, KVV Prasad and Niveditha H. Public oral primary preventive measures: An Indian perspective. JIOH Volume 3; Issue 5: October 2011.7-18.

Uwayezu D, Gatarayiha A and Nzayirambaho M. Prevalence of dental caries and associated risk factors in children living with disabilities in Rwanda: a cross-sectional study. Pan Afr Med J. 2020 Jul 17; 36:193.

WHO Oral Health Country/Area Profile Project, WHO Collaborating Centre, Malmö University, Sweden.

World Health Organization, 2009. Global Data on Dental Caries Prevalence (DMFT) in Children Aged 12 years. Global Oral Data Bank. Oral health country/area profile programme, Management of noncommunicable diseases. Geneva, May 2000. WHO/NMH/MNC/ORH/Caries.12y.00.3.

World Health Organization. Oral Health Promotion: An Essential Element of a Health-Promoting School. WHO Information Series on School Health (Document Eleven). WHO, Geneva, 2003. WHO/NMH/NPH/ORH/School/03.3.

CHAPTER 9

Dental Plaque

HIGHLIGHTS

- Plaque contains millions of bacteria, which can cause gum disease and tooth decay if left unchecked.
- Back then, the notion held that dental diseases were caused by an excess of all the microorganisms present in dental plaque.
- The processes that lead to dental plaque production include bacterial colonization, biofilm formation, sticky film formation, mineralization, and maturation.
- As plaque ages and mineralizes, cavities form, causing irritation, resorption, and eventual tooth loss.
- Good oral hygiene practices, such as brushing, flossing, controlling one's diet, giving up smoking, and getting regular dental exams, all help to avoid dental plaque.

Dental plaque is a continuously forming layer of bacteria that is soft, sticky, colourless, or pale yellow on the teeth and gums. It is a biofilm made up of saliva, bacteria, and their waste products. When oral bacteria interact with the sugars and starches in our diet, plaque is created. Plaque can build up and harden into tartar, also known as dental calculus, if it is not eliminated by consistent and efficient oral hygiene procedures like brushing and flossing. Tartar is more difficult to remove and can be a factor in a number of dental issues, such as gum disease and tooth decay. Tartar removal and maintaining oral health often require routine dental cleanings. Dental plaque forms via an ordered sequence of events, resulting in a structurally- and functionally-organized, species-rich microbial community (Marsh, 2004). Distinct stages in plaque formation include: acquired pellicle formation; reversible adhesion involving weak long-range physico-chemical interactions between the cell surface and the pellicle, which can lead to stronger adhesin-receptor mediated attachment; co-adhesion resulting in attachment of secondary colonizers to already attached cells; multiplication and biofilm formation (including the synthesis of exopolysaccharides) and, on occasion, detachment (Kolenbrander *et al*., 2000). Saliva, sugars, acids, germs, and food particles mix to form a soft, sticky film on teeth within 20 minutes of eating. Dental plaque can form anywhere in the mouth, although it usually gathers in the deep fissures surrounding the molars.

9.1. History of Dental Plaque formation

Antonie van Leeuwenhoek noted dental plaque for the first time in the 17th century, and he connected it to prevalent dental conditions. At the time, the theory put forth was that tooth illnesses resulted from an overabundance of every microbe found in dental plaque. The hypothesis was the subject of debate for more than a century. This theory, known as the nonspecific plaque hypothesis (NSPH), was based on the amount of plaque that indicated pathogenicity without taking the virulence of the different microorganisms into account. According to the aspects of Evolution, dental plaque has existed throughout human existence. The shift from a hunter-gatherer to an agriculturist lifestyle was accompanied by dietary changes, especially the addition of additional carbohydrates, which increased the prevalence of dental plaque and associated oral health problems. Archaeological research provides evidence that ancient societies maintained some sort of dental hygiene. Teeth were cleaned with sticks that were ragged or twigs. In certain societies, teeth were cleaned using abrasive powders created from materials like crushed bones and oyster shells. The teeth-cleaning techniques employed by the ancient Greeks and Romans included the use of toothpicks and a variety of cleaning solutions. Oral hygiene procedures were not as sophisticated as they are now, though. Controlling dental plaque has advanced significantly with the invention of toothbrushes and toothpaste in more recent times, as well as a greater knowledge of the role of bacteria in oral health. Dental research is still being done today to find solutions for managing and preventing dental plaque.

9.2. Nature of Dental Plaque

The process of dental plaque production begins with the colonization of bacteria, primarily *Streptococcus mutans*, however other species of bacteria can also contribute to the formation of dental plaque. These microorganisms break down the sugars and starches in our meals to produce acids that can damage dental enamel. A complex community of microorganisms embedded in a matrix of extracellular polymeric substances (EPS) is what is known as a plaque. The bacteria are shielded from mechanical removal and antibacterial agents by this matrix. When food particles contact with bacteria that have colonized the tooth surfaces, plaque is created. A sticky film is formed by the bacteria's attachment to the teeth and to one another. Dental calculus, often known as tartar, can occur as plaque ages and mineralizes if it is not removed. Tartar is a more resilient material that is more challenging to eliminate and offers a surface

9.3. Prime reasons for plaque

It is inevitable for teeth to develop plaque. This is due to the fact that oral bacteria consume everything we eat for growth and survival. While the bacteria prefer sweet and starchy carbohydrates, they also take what they require from other foods. These bacteria eventually create acids, which erode tooth enamel over time. Additionally, they result in cavities, or holes in the teeth, which are the initial indications of dental decay. Additionally, plaque can form behind the gum line, weakening the bone that supports the tooth.

9.4. Complications of Dental plaque

Accumulation of dental plaque can lead to gingivitis (inflammation of the gums and soft tissues in the oral cavity) and also periodontitis. Early stages of infection of this sort are limited to inflammation of the oral soft tissues (gingivitis) and do not leave traces in the bone. With advanced cases that progress to periodontitis, the periodontal ligaments and alveolus become involved and it is at this point that the disease can be observed in skeletal remains. Generally, the infection progresses into the gomphosis of the tooth and affects the periodontal ligaments holding the tooth in place. The resulting inflammation, accumulation of plaque, and loss of periodontal attachment result in alveolar bone resorption and loss (Hillson, 2000). This loss is most often found in the molars and ultimately presents as a recession of the alveolus and exposure of the root. The surface of the alveolus may present as porotic and may extend beyond a single tooth. Affected teeth may be loose in their sockets due to the bone resorption and loss of periodontal ligaments. Standards for the recording of periodontal disease can be found in Hildebolt and Molnar (1991). Michalowicz and colleagues (2000) estimate a heritability rate of 50% based on their study of twins. This indicates that earlier studies that had reported variation in prevalence between populations attributed to hygiene differences (Loe et al., 1992) may have overlooked the underlying genetic predisposition to periodontal disease.

9.5. An overview of the creation of plaque in childhood

Infants can acquire bacteria linked to dental plaque from their caretakers. Sharing cutlery or wiping pacifiers with saliva are common examples of this. The mouth cavity starts to become colonized by microorganisms. When kids start eating solid foods, particularly those high in sugars and starches, oral bacteria feed on these substances and produce acids that aid in the development of plaque. Plaque can grow on teeth after prolonged contact to sugary beverages from bottles or sippy cups, such as fruit juices or formula. This may be a factor in dental decay in young children, or caries. Primary (baby) tooth eruption produces more surfaces on which plaque can accumulate.

First and foremost, parents are the primary caregivers for young children when it comes to dental hygiene. To clean the gums and erupting teeth, they could use a tiny, soft toothbrush or a gentle cloth. When more teeth erupt, brushing should be done using a child-friendly toothbrush and a tiny dab of fluoride toothpaste (as advised by dental professionals). Until a kid reaches the age of seven or eight, or until they have the manual skill to brush well, parents should monitor their use of a toothbrush. Establishing the groundwork for lifelong healthy dental habits in children begins with teaching them the value of dental hygiene, which includes brushing and flossing on a regular basis. Before turning one year old or six months after their first tooth erupts, children should see a dentist for the first time. Frequent dental examinations make it possible to identify and treat dental problems early on. Early childhood caries can be avoided by limiting the use of sugary foods and beverages. Using fluoride can improve tooth enamel and lower the risk of cavities, whether it is administered professionally or through toothpaste.

9.6. Dental Plaque Prevention Techniques

A healthy diet, frequent dental checkups, and proper oral hygiene habits all contribute to the prevention of dental plaque. The following are important methods for avoiding dental plaque:

- **Brushing:** Brush teeth twice a day, ideally in the morning and right before bed. Apply fluoride toothpaste and a toothbrush with soft bristles. Avoid the brush chewing, rear, and front surfaces of teeth. Every three to four months, or sooner if the bristles are frayed, replace toothbrush.
- **Flossing:** Use dental floss to get rid of dirt and plaque from places that toothbrush could miss. The right way to use floss is to gently move it between each tooth and along the gum line. Do not snap the floss; this can cause damage to our gums.
- **Use of Antibacterial Mouthwash**: This help lessen oral bacteria, use an antimicrobial or antibacterial mouthwash.
- **Reduce Sugary Food Consumption**: Eat less starchy and sugary foods because they can aggravate plaque development. Acids produced by oral bacteria as a result of feeding on sweets can cause tooth decay. For overall dental and general health, maintain a diet rich in fruits, vegetables, whole grains, and lean meats.
- **Water Intake:** Throughout the day, sip a lot of water. Water facilitates the removal of microorganisms and food particles from the mouth, creating a healthier environment.
- **Frequent dental examinations:** Make time for routine dental cleanings and examinations. Professional cleanings get rid of tartar and plaque that routine brushing and flossing might not be able to. By scheduling routine dental examinations, dental problems can be identified and treated before they worsen.
- **Avoid Smoking:** Giving Up tobacco usage or smoking might enhance your oral health and lower your chance of developing problems with plaque.

Instruct kids and family members on the value of maintaining proper oral hygiene practices and how they can help to avoid dental plaque. We can greatly lower your risk of dental plaque development and associated oral health problems by adopting these habits into your daily life and scheduling routine dental examinations.

References

Becky De Spain Eden. Preventive Strategies Directed Toward Microbial Agents. Prevention in Clinical Oral Health Care, 2008.

Dina G. Moussa, Paras Ahmad, Tamer A. Mansour, and Walter L. Siqueira. Current state and challenges of the global outcome of dental caries research. Front. Cell Infect. Microbiol. 2022. (12). 1-23.

Karygianni, L, Karygianni, Z. Ren, H. Koo,and T. Thurnheer, Z. Ren, H. Koo, and T. Thurnheer. Biofilm Matrixome: Extracellular Components in Structured Microbial Communities. Trends in Microbiology, August 2020, Vol. 28, No. 8 669.

Philip D Marsh. Dental plaque as a biofilm and a microbial community – implications for health and disease. Biotechnology and Biomaterials to Reduce the Caries Epidemic. BMC Oral Health 2006, 6: S14.

Online Resources

https://www.byte.com/community/resources/article/do-dont-brushing-teeth/

https://www.ancientpages.com/2015/12/26/ancient-egyptians-invented-toothpaste/

HIGHLIGHTS

- The human heart is a vital organ that pumps blood throughout the body, removes waste, and supplies oxygen and sustenance to tissues and organs.
- The development of IE has been linked to a number of bacteria, 90% of which are either stable or transitory members of the oral microbiota.
- As a result, IE is believed to be among the most prevalent chronic inflammatory illnesses in adults, with a prevalence that rises with age and corresponds with the age at which patients present with IE.
- The prophylactic use of antibiotics, coagulation targeting, good dental hygiene, and antibiofilm therapy are the strategies used to prevent IE.

CHAPTER 10

Dental Caries V/S Infective Endocarditis

The Heart wall is composed of three layers, including the outer epicardium (thin layer), middle myocardium (thick layer), and innermost endocardium (thin layer). The myocardium is made up of cardiac muscle fibers and is responsible for the contraction and relaxation that results in the pumping of the heart. The two atria have a thinner myocardium layer than the ventricles, as the force required for atrial contractions is much less than that needed for ventricular contractions. The walls of the right ventricle are also thinner, as this ventricle only pumps blood a short distance to the lungs. Comparatively, the left ventricle, which has much thicker walls, must generate enough force to pump oxygenated blood throughout the rest of the body.

The myocardium requires a constant supply of oxygen and nutrients to maintain the contractions and relaxations that keep the heart pumping. This blood supply is maintained through a set of coronary arteries and veins in the myocardium. The right and left coronary arteries, which branch off the first section of the aorta known as the ascending aorta between the left ventricle and aortic arch, supply blood to a network of capillaries in the myocardium. Deoxygenated blood from the myocardium is carried through a set of cardiac veins to the right atrium that is subsequently drained through the coronary sinus.

10.1. Cardiovascular Diseases

Heart-related problems that are frequently seen include cardiovascular disorders, which include arrhythmias, heart failure, and coronary artery disease. Valve malformations and diseases result in a staggering number of deaths each year. Stenosis, which is the obstructed outflow of blood and regurgitation or backward flow of blood due to defective closure of valves, are manifestations of valve diseases. Heart sounds are caused by vibrations produced during the closure of valves. Abnormal heart sounds, or heart murmurs, indicate valve malfunctions.

The most common valve malformations include the bicuspid aortic valve and mitral valve prolapse. Valve disease can also occur through the degeneration of elastin, collagen, and proteoglycan layers of the extracellular matrix of the valves. Coronary heart diseases (CHD) or ischemic heart diseases progress slowly. They are caused by atherosclerosis, or the buildup of fat, cholesterol, or calcium on the walls of the coronary arteries that supply blood to the heart. This results in a reduced supply of oxygenated blood to the heart. Pieces of these fat deposits can also break off, forming a blood clot that can block the coronary artery, cut off blood supply to the heart, and cause a heart attack. Symptoms of CHD include chest pain, nausea, traveling pain through the limbs, and shortness of breath. High blood pressure, smoking, high cholesterol, diabetes, and obesity are risk factors for CHD.

10.2. Infective endocarditis (IE)

Infective endocarditis (IE) is a devastating cardiovascular disease originated by an inflammation of the endocardium, heart valves, atria, and ventricles walls (Carinci et al., 2018). Despite its low incidence, the comprehensive armamentarium of antimicrobial therapy, improved surgical intervention techniques, prognosis and the overall mortality rate remain high (in hospital 3-month mortality is about 20%) (Lung & Duval, 2019). IE is often caused by either bacteria or other microorganisms like viruses and fungi. The colonization of the endocardium is a complex process that typically starts with the adherence of microorganisms in susceptible valves. The development of endocarditis requires a complex interplay of different factors that cause certain microorganisms to adhere to the cardiac endothelium and trigger an inflammatory process. Congenital or acquired diseases of the heart can lead to partial loss of endothelial integrity, resulting in an increased risk for the development of infective endocarditis (Wilson *et al.,* 2007).

Loss of endothelial integrity and disruption of the inner cell layer enable the formation of a platelet-derived thrombus and a corresponding inflammatory cascade. The resulting non-bacterial endocarditis (NBTE) is considered a prerequisite for the adhesion of microorganisms that enter the bloodstream in the course of bacteraemia (Moreillon *et al.*, 1988).

10.3. Oral Microbiota and the Pathogenesis of Infective Endocarditis (IE)

The cause of transient bacteraemia usually lies in the disintegration of a bacterially colonized surface, such as the skin or mucous membrane, which harbours numerous commensals but also opportunistic pathogens. While up to 90% of IE are caused by gram-positive *Staphylococcus sp.* (species), *Streptococcus sp.* and *Enterococcus sp.* (Cahill & Prendergast, 2016), Staphylococcus aureus is considered the most common in high-income countries (Selton-Suty *et al.*, 2012). Coagulase-negative *Staphylococcus sp.* such as *Staphylococcus epidermis* are ubiquitous skin commensals and account for approximately 10% of IE whereas streptococcal infections by the oral viridans group (e.g., *S. mutans*, *S. mitis*, *S. anguinis*) cause almost 20% of infective endocarditis (Cahill & Prendergast, 2016). Hence, a more precise evaluation of the oral cavity as an outstanding environment for bacteria is reasonable. The oral microbiome consists of over 700 different species of bacteria (Palmer, 2012), including numerous commensals and also opportunistic pathogens, some of which are organized in complex biofilms entering the bloodstream in the event of mucosal or gingival disruption. Traumatic injury to the mucosa or gingiva as part of physiological processes such as chewing food or oral hygiene (Lockhart *et al.,* 2009), but also particularly in diseases such as dental caries or periodontitis and their secondary symptoms, as well as in various therapeutic measures for their prevention and treatment, can thus inevitably lead to the transfer of bacterial pathogens from the oral cavity into the bloodstream, resulting in bacteremia. Bacterial adhesion of microorganisms to disrupted endothelial walls and resulting thrombotic formations is promoted by specific mediators such as surface components that serve as virulence factors in various microbial species (Moreillon *et al.*, 2002). In this manner, several species of streptococci, staphylococci and enterococci can colonize impaired endocardium and cause infective endocarditis.

Several clinical studies have demonstrated that routine activities such as flossing, tooth brushing, and chewing may cause gingival bleeding and are responsible for a higher number of circulating bacteria, daily (Lockhart *et al.*, 2008). In addition, more invasive procedures such as endodontic procedures, tooth extractions, elimination of caries concerning cervical or subgingival portions of the tooth, periodontal and apical surgery, may induce gingival or mucosal traumas, causing transient bacteraemia (Dajani *et al.*, 1987). Importantly the healthy cardiac endothelium mostly unaffected by this form of bacteremia, although this is even more extensive than that due to an invasive procedure (Lockhart *et al.,* 2008). However, starting in 1955, the American Heart Association recommended the use of antibiotics to reduce the risk of IE in patients with underlying cardiac conditions undergoing bacteraemia-producing procedures, with a great emphasis on dental procedures (Jones *et al.*, 1995).

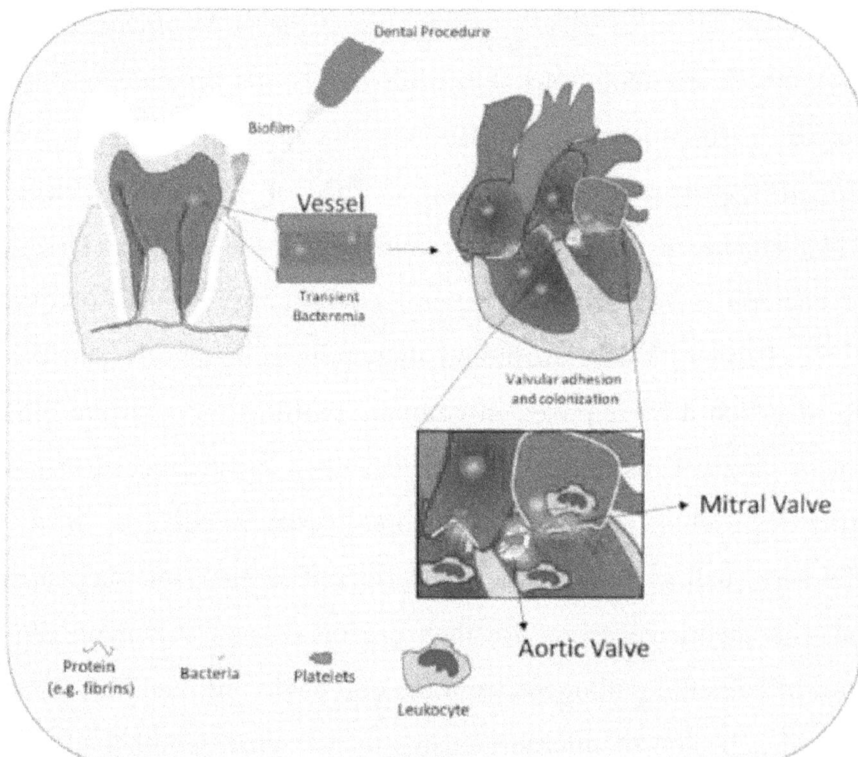

Different stages of endocarditis development after dental procedures

10.4. Prevalence of Infective endocarditis

It is the second-most diffused oral disease and the sixth disease most diffused globally, affecting more than 746,000,000 people around the world, according to a recent meta-regression by the Global Burden of Disease study on more than 290,000 subjects (Kassebaum *et al.,* 2014). Indeed, the prevalence of moderate and severe periodontitis amounts to 42% and 11%, respectively (Eke *et al.*, 2000). However, the distribution of this, and of other oral diseases, shows a steep increase after the second decade of life, with the prevalence reaching the highest values in the elderly (Martu *et al.,* 2000). Hence, it is thought to be one of the most common chronic inflammatory diseases in adults with an age-rising prevalence matching with the increasing age of patients presenting IE (Cecchi *et al.,* 2015. This disease is often caused by an alteration of symbiotic oral microbiota, with significant proliferation of Gram-negative bacteria described as periodontal pathogenssuch as *Porphyromonas gingivalis* (P. gingivalis), an anaerobic pathogen, that can determine loss of dental attachment (Liccardo *et al.*, 2019). Subsequently, the sulcular epithelium begins to ulcerate, allowing the microorganisms to enter the bloodstream (Liccardo *et al.,* 2019). Based on this premise, for years, antibiotic prophylaxis strategies have been proposed for patients with IE to reduce the risk related to dental or other procedures determining bacteremia (Jones *et al.,* 1995). However, strategies still have contrasting opinions, as the proof of their efficacy is lacking, and as there is the demonstration that oral bacteremia, able to influence IE, may occur after daily procedures such as toothbrushing, flossing, or chewing (Patini *et al.,* 2018).

10.5. Prevention of Infective Endocarditis

The American Heart Association in 1955 recommended the use of antibiotics to reduce the risk of IE in patients with underlying cardiac conditions undergoing bacteraemia-producing procedures (Jones et al., 1995). The recommendations were based on IE animal models and in vitro susceptibilities of microorganisms known to cause endocarditis. Amoxicillin has been shown to significantly impact the incidence and duration of bacteremia after dental procedures (Lockhart *et al.*, 2004). Since then, several updates of the guidelines have taken place. The great debate raised around antibiotic prophylaxis asks for new innovative therapies. In this scenario, the coagulation system appears as a novel potential and attractive therapeutic target. Indeed, IE is one of the best-characterized clinical models, where infection, inflammation, and coagulation are strongly interconnected in a bidirectional relationship which is often referred to as immunothrombosis (Que & Moreillon, 2011). The interactions between pathogens and platelets and the activation of the coagulation system are critical to initiation and growth of vegetation (Durante-Mangoni *et al.*, 2014). Thus, preventing this procoagulant imbalance with antiplatelet and anticoagulant strategies would represent a valid cornerstone of IE management.

The improvement to high levels of oral hygiene and their maintenance should be considered from an oral health standpoint and possibly reduce the risk of IE. However, for a proper reduction of dental plaque, regular oral hygiene procedures should be completed with interdental cleaning devices. While flossing was previously considered the gold standard, inter-dental brushes seem to be more effective (Kotsakis *et al.,* 2018). The use of biofilm eradication agents that comprise a variety of promising molecules (i.e., antimicrobial Peptides, Quaternary ammonium compounds, antimicrobial lipids) offers exciting prospects for the future of biofilm therapeutics, especially for those infections that are refractory to conventional antibiotics (Arciola *et al.,* 2014).

Since its initial description more than 130 years ago, infective endocarditis has been the focus of study. The first clinical guidelines for the prevention of IE were published in the 1950s by the American Heart Association (AHA), emphasizing dental procedures and antibiotic prophylaxis. Since then, guidelines and updates for the prevention of infective endocarditis have been published by the American Heart Association, the European Society of Cardiology (ESC), and a number of other national and international societies. These updates include recommendations regarding the necessity of antibiotic prophylaxis prior to dental procedures. On whether these preventive suggestions can be effectively implemented, however, there is still disagreement, particularly with regard to patients with congenital heart abnormalities (CHD).

References

Bumm CV, Folwaczny M. Infective endocarditis and oral health-a Narrative Review. Cardiovasc Diagn Ther. 2021 Dec;11(6):1403-1415. doi: 10.21037/cdt-20-908.

Carinci F., Martinelli M., Contaldo M., Santoro R., Pezzetti F., Lauritano D., Candotto V., Mucchi D., Palmieri A., Tagliabue A., et al. Focus on periodontal disease and development of endocarditis. Biol. Regul. Homeost. Agents. 2018; 32:143–147.

Cecchi E., Chirillo F., Castiglione A., Faggiano P., Cecconi M., Moreo A., Cialfi A., Rinaldi M., Del Ponte S., Squeri A., et al. Clinical epidemiology in Italian Registry of Infective Endocarditis (RIEI): Focus on age, intravascular devices and enterococci. Int. J. Cardiol. 2015; 190:151–156. doi: 10.1016/j.ijcard.2015.04.123.

Christine Selton-Suty , Marie Célard, Vincent Le Moing, et al. Preeminence of Staphylococcus aureus in infective endocarditis: a 1-year population-based survey. Clin Infect Dis. 2012 May;54(9):1230-9. doi: 10.1093/cid/cis199.

Del Giudice C, Vaia E, Liccardo D, Marzano F, Valletta A, Spagnuolo G, Ferrara N,

Eke P.I., Borgnakke W.S., Genco R.J. Recent epidemiologic trends in periodontitis in the USA. Periodontology 2000. 2020; 82:257–267. doi: 10.1111/prd.12323.

Hinton RB, Yutzey KE. Heart valve structure and function in development and disease. Annu Rev Physiol. 2011; 73:29-46.

Jones, T. D, L. Baumgartner, M.T. Bellows, *et al.*Prevention of rheumatic fever and bacterial endocarditis through control of streptococcal infections Circulation, 11 (1955), pp. 317-320.

Liccardo D., Marzano F., Carraturo F., Guida M., Femminella G.D., Bencivenga L., Agrimi J., Addonizio A., Melino I., Valletta A., et al. Potential bidirectional relationship between periodontitis and Alzheimer's Disease. Front. Physiol. 2020; 11:683–695. doi: 10.3389/fphys.2020.00683.

Lockhart, P.B, M.T. Brennan, M. Thornhill, *et al.* Poor oral hygiene as a risk factor for infective endocarditis-related bacteremia. J Am Dent Assoc, 140 (2009), pp. 1238-1244.

Martu M.A., Maftei G.A., Luchian I., Popa C., Filioreanu A.M., Tatarciuc D., Nichitean G., Hurjui L.L., Foia L.G. Wound healing of periodontal and oral tissues: Part II—Patho-phisiological conditions and metabolic diseases. Rom. J. Oral Rehab. 2020; 12:30–40.

Patini R., Gallenzi P., Spagnuolo G., Cordaro M., Cantiani M., Amalfitano A., Arcovito A., Callà C., Mingrone G., Nocca G. Correlation Between Metabolic Syndrome, Periodontitis and Reactive Oxygen Species Production. A Pilot Study. Open Dent. J. 2017; 11:621–627. doi: 10.2174/1874210601711010621

Rengo C, Cannavo A, Rengo G. Infective Endocarditis: A Focus on Oral Microbiota.

Thomas J Cahill , Larry M Baddour , Gilbert Habib , Bruno Hoen , Erwan Salaun· Gosta B Pettersson , Hans Joachim Schäfers , Bernard D Prendergast. Challenges in Infective Endocarditis. J Am Coll Cardiol. 2016 ;69(3): 325-344.doi: 10.1016/j.jacc.2016.10.066.

Walter Wilson , Kathryn A Taubert, et al. Prevention of infective endocarditis: guidelines from the American Heart Association. Circulation. 2007 Oct 9;116(15):1736-54. doi: 10.1161/CIRCULATIONAHA.106.183095.

Yok-Ai Que , Philippe Moreillon. Infective endocarditis. Nat Rev Cardiol. 2011 Jun;8(6):322-36. doi: 10.1038/nrcardio.2011.43.

CHAPTER 11

Dental Caries V/S Alzheimer's

HIGHLIGHTS

- Science still doesn't know what causes Alzheimer's disease in most cases.
- These plaques and tangles in the brain are still thought to be some of the main signs and symptoms of Alzheimer's.
- The early-onset stage of Alzheimer's disease affects persons between the ages of thirty and sixty-five in less than 10% of instances.
- According to a recent study conducted by experts at NIA, dementia, especially Alzheimer's disease, is linked to the bacteria that cause gum disease.
- When it comes to providing care for an Alzheimer's patient, prevention is essential. Give them clear, concise instructions, such as to clean their teeth at least twice a day.

Alzheimer's disease is a neurological condition that worsens over time and damages the brain, causing memory loss, cognitive decline, and ultimately the inability to carry out daily duties. Although the precise causation of Alzheimer's disease is unknown, a mix of genetic, environmental, and lifestyle factors are thought to be involved. Symptoms usually include memory loss, disorientation, trouble solving problems, and personality or mood swings. As the illness worsens, people may get disoriented, struggle to speak, and find it difficult to carry out daily duties. The majority of people's cause of Alzheimer's disease is still unknown to science. The elements listed above are most likely a combination of the reasons. Depending on the individual, each of these characteristics may have varying effects on the likelihood of developing Alzheimer's disease. Alzheimer's is typically thought of as a progressive brain illness. It is typified by alterations in the brain, such as the formation of neurofibrillary tangles, also known as tau plaques, and amyloid plaques, which cause neurons and their connections to die. A person's memory, cognitive function, and ultimately their capacity to live independently are all impacted by these and other changes. Dr. Alois Alzheimer is the namesake of Alzheimer's disease. Dr. Alzheimer observed alterations in the brain tissue of a woman who passed away from an uncommon mental condition in 1906. Her symptoms included erratic conduct, memory loss, and linguistic issues. He studied her brain after she passed away and discovered several aberrant clusters, which are now known as amyloid plaques, and twisted fiber bundles, which are known as neurofibrillary, or tau, tangles. These brain tangles and plaques are still regarded as some of the primary characteristics of Alzheimer's. The loss of neuronal connections in the brain is another characteristic. Neurons are responsible for sending messages from the brain to the body's muscles and organs as well as within the brain itself.

Alzheimer's disease is a brain ailment that gradually impairs thinking and memory abilities as well as the capacity to do even the most basic duties. The majority of Alzheimer's patients experience symptoms later in life. The severity of dementia varies, with the least severe stage occurring when a person's functioning is just starting to be affected and the most severe stage necessitating total reliance on others for assistance with daily activities. Depending on the kinds of brain alterations that may be occurring, dementia can have a variety of causes. Lewy body dementia, frontotemporal diseases, and vascular dementia are among the other types of dementia. People with mixed dementia, which combines two or more kinds of dementia, are not uncommon. Brain alterations may start ten years or more before symptoms manifest. The brain is undergoing harmful alterations in this extremely early stage of Alzheimer's disease, including aberrant protein accumulations that result in tau tangles and amyloid plaques. Previously healthy neurons eventually die, stop working, and lose their connections to other neurons. Alzheimer's disease is also believed to be influenced by a wide range of other intricate brain abnormalities. The entorhinal cortex and the hippocampal regions, which are crucial for memory formation, appear to be the first areas of the brain to sustain injury. More areas of the brain become damaged and start to shrink as more neurons die. Brain tissue has greatly shrunk and there has been extensive damage by the time Alzheimer's reaches its last stage.

Beyond the age of 65, the number of cases of Alzheimer's disease about doubles every five years. Approximately one-third of adults over 85 may develop Alzheimer's disease. These age-related alterations include the atrophy (shrinking) of specific brain regions, vascular damage, inflammation, the release of unstable chemicals known as free radicals, and a breakdown in the cells' ability to produce energy. Many people are afraid they will develop Alzheimer's, especially if a family member has already been affected by the disease. Just because someone in family has had the sickness in the past does not mean that person will acquire it as well. On the other hand, it could suggest a greater chance of developing it. Genes inherited from one's biological parents can impact an individual's genetic susceptibility to Alzheimer's disease. Alzheimer's disease has two types: early-onset and late-onset. Both have a genetic component.

11.1 Risk factor for the Alzheimer's

The late-onset type of the disease is not directly caused by a single gene, according to research. Having one allele of the apolipoprotein E (APOE) gene on chromosome 19 increases a person's risk, however it is only one genetic risk factor. Nonetheless, the presence of the APOE □4 allele does not guarantee the development of Alzheimer's. While some individuals with an APOE ε4 allele never get Alzheimer's, others who do have the illness have no APOE ς4 alleles. The goal of research is to find more genetic risk variations for Alzheimer's disease that develops slowly. Less than 10% of cases of Alzheimer's disease are early-onset, occurring in adults between the ages of thirty and sixty-five. Numerous variables other than genetics could contribute to the onset and progression of Alzheimer's disease. For instance, there is a lot of interest in the connection between metabolic disorders like diabetes and obesity and vascular diseases like high blood pressure, heart disease, and stroke, as well as cognitive loss. Early-life circumstances could also be important. For instance, research has shown a lower risk of dementia with more educational attainment. Additionally, research is being done to better understand the origins of Alzheimer's disease and to find effective therapies and preventions for everyone. There are disparities in dementia risk among sexes and racial groups.

11.2. Development of Alzheimer’s disease due to Poor oral health

According to a recent review by NIA scientists published in the Journal of Alzheimer's Disease, bacteria that cause gum disease may also have a role in the emergence of Alzheimer's disease and other related dementias, including vascular dementia. An infection of the oral tissues that hold teeth in place is the cause of gum disease. The primary symptoms of this illness are bleeding gums, loose teeth, and even tooth loss. Through the bloodstream, bacteria and the inflammatory chemicals they produce can spread from oral infections to the brain. A team from the National Centre for Health Statistics and the National Health and Nutrition Examination Survey (NHANES) conducted at a sizable population study on dental conditions associated with dementia. The study included almost 6,000 people in various age groups at baseline and followed them for up to 26 years. In order to determine if antibodies against 19 oral bacteria are associated with Alzheimer's disease diagnosis, dementia diagnosis of any kind, or Alzheimer's disease death, the team analysed the antibodies. When gum disease occurs, *Porphyromonas gingivalis* is the most common cause. In fact, a new study hypothesizes that this infection may cause the production of beta-amyloid protein plaques, a significant hallmark of Alzheimer's disease.

This ecosystem is in a fragile balance to maintain oral health. In healthy conditions, Gram-positive bacteria dominate the composition of the dental plaque. However, because of different factors such as sugars, acids, or a lack of tooth brushing, the plaque composition could evolve into having a greater proportion of Gram-negative anaerobic bacteria (Masson, 2021). This altered balance, also named oral dysbiosis, can lead to oral pathologies such as periodontal disease (PD). The inflammation, which starts in the gum area, is called gingivitis. When the gum inflammation persists and progresses, it creates the conditions for the development of periodontitis (Pizzo *et al.,* 2010), which can spread to the alveolar bone, the cementum, and the periodontal ligament. The periodonto pathogenic bacteria inflammation mediators and toxins, which go into the bloodstream and participate in systemic inflammation. Consequently, chronic periodontitis can contribute to the development of various pathologies (Kurgan and Kantarci, 2018).

Researchers at the School of Dentistry, University of Central Lancashire (UCLan), were the first to report the link between gum disease and Alzheimer's disease. Marking this important awareness day, (World Alzheimer's Month and 21 September) the two new studies give a better understanding of the defining Alzheimer's disease lesions on the brain: technically known as amyloid-beta plaques and neurofibrillary tangles. The exact cause of this disease is not yet fully understood, which means it's a difficult disease to prevent and treat. The first study, being published in the *Journal of Alzheimer's Disease*, shows that nerve cells in the brain contain a type of protein called tau. When tau meets the gingipains enzyme, the tau releases from the nerve cell. Once freed, tau physically changes, in the form of coils and non-coiling filaments. These filaments of tau then re-attach to the nerve cell and become incorporated into the lesion known as neurofibrillary tangles. These ultimately kill the nerve cells. What this means is that once a nerve cell dies and the free tau protein leaks into the brain, the tau may attach itself to healthy neighbouring nerve cells, repeating the process and leading to further damage to the brain as the disease spreads (Kanagasingam *et al.,* 2022).

The second study, published in the *Journal of Alzheimer's Disease Reports*, looks at the way the gingipains enzyme, released by the bacterium, can contribute to the formation of amyloid-beta plaques - another of the lesions, alongside the tangles, which form on the brains of those suffering from Alzheimer's. These studies are small steps in the fight against Alzheimer's, but the results are significant in understanding the role of gingipains and how fundamental they are to lesion formation. It is hoped that studies such as these will help with developing future treatments. Shalini Kanagasingam, Specialist Endodontist and Senior Clinical Lecturer at UCLan, who led the study (supervised by Dr Sim K. Singhrao) said: 'What this kind of research proves is the importance of our oral health. Look out for early signs of gum disease such as bleeding gums when brushing or more advanced signs like movement or drifting of the teeth. Don't delay or skip your dental check-ups. Your dentist will be able to help advise you on how to effectively remove plaque and tartar from your teeth, which harbour the bacterium that we have identified as a risk factor for Alzheimer's. These studies highlight the key message that a healthy mouth is important for maintaining a healthy body and mind' (Kanagasingam *et al.,* 2022).

11.3. Caring for an Alzheimer's Patient's Oral Health

Patients that have Alzheimer's disease typically experience worsening oral health as their condition progresses. In the earlier stages of the disease, patients can often continue their daily routines — including brushing their teeth and getting to the dentist. As their condition worsens and their cognitive function decreases, Alzheimer's patients forget these routines that they may have had their entire life. This can have detrimental effects on their oral health and overall wellbeing. Prevention is vital when it comes to caring for a patient with Alzheimer's. Offer short and simple directions includes help brush their teeth at least twice a day, demonstrate how to brush properly, try different toothbrushes to see which works best, Find the right dentist to care for their needs, Stay aware of any discomfort or pain in the mouth, Properly sanitize dentures Keep a record of recent dental appointments.

References

Azheimer's Disease a Much Larger Cause of Death Than Previously Recognized. Available from: https://www.rush.edu/news/alzheimers-disease-much-larger-cause-death previously-recognized (accessed February 28, 2021).

Cummings JL, Morstorf T, and Zhong K. Alzheimer's disease drug-development pipeline: few candidates, frequent failures. *Alzheimers Res Ther.* (2014) 6:37. doi: 10.1186/alzrt269

Facts and Figures. *Alzheimer's Disease and Dementia.* Available from: https://www.alz.org/alzheimers-dementia/facts-figures (accessed February 28, 2021).

Kanagasingam S, Chukkapalli SS, Welbury R, and Singhrao SK. Porphyromonas gingivalis is a strong risk factor for Alzheimer's disease. J Alzheimers Dis Rep. (2020) 4:501–11. doi: 10.3233/ADR-200250.

Kurgan S., Kantarci A. Molecular Basis for Immunohistochemical and Inflammatory Changes during Progression of Gingivitis to Periodontitis. *Periodontol 2000.* 2018;**76**:51–67. doi: 10.1111/prd.12146.

Masson E. Le Microbiote Buccal: Bases Fondamentales et Applications en Physiopathologie.

Pizzo G., Guiglia R., Lo Russo L., Campisi G. Dentistry and Internal Medicine: From the Focal Infection Theory to the Periodontal Medicine Concept. *Eur. J. Intern. Med.* 2010; 21:496–502. doi: 10.1016/j.ejim.2010.07.011.

CHAPTER

12

Oral Health V/S Cerebrovascular Accident

HIGHLIGHTS

- The human brain is a very complex organ that is essential to the control of numerous bodily functions as well as mental processes.
- A cerebrovascular accident (CVA), commonly referred to as a stroke, is brought on by a partial or complete blockage of blood supply to the brain.
- Studies using epidemiology have looked into the connections between stroke and dental conditions. There seems to be an oblique or circumstantial connection here.
- One of these microorganisms, Streptococcus mutant, is critical for the earlier development of stroke in both haemorrhagic stroke patients and rats.
- Early research revealed an increased risk of damage from a quiet stroke in those with a genetic predisposition to cavities, missing teeth, or requiring dentures.

The human brain is an extremely intricate organ that is crucial to the regulation of many body systems and mental activities. The brain's ability to operate properly depends on blood flow because blood purges waste materials from the body while delivering nutrients and oxygen. The cerebral circulation is the network of blood arteries that supplies blood to the brain. The vertebral arteries and the left and right internal carotid arteries are the two main blood vessels that deliver blood to the brain. Even in the event that an artery becomes blocked, the Circle of Willis, a network of connecting arteries at the base of the brain, helps guarantee a continuous blood flow to the brain. Red blood cells carry oxygen, which is necessary for the brain's metabolic functions. To supply energy for the brain's functions, the blood also carries nutrients, including glucose. The brain is remarkably adept at controlling blood flow to satisfy its own metabolic needs. We refer to this mechanism as brain autoregulation. The dilation or constriction of blood arteries in the brain to maintain a stable blood flow is influenced by various factors, including variations in blood pressure, carbon dioxide levels, and cerebral activity. Disorders that impact cerebral blood flow might have serious repercussions. Examples include disorders affecting the blood vessels (e.g., aneurysms, arteriosclerosis) and stroke (caused by a shortage of blood supply to portion of the brain). A stroke is a process in which blood flow to the brain is suddenly interrupted. When the brain does not receive enough blood supply, it may result in permanent brain cell damage. Strokes can take two forms. A stroke, also known as a cerebrovascular accident (CVA), is caused by a partial or total obstruction of blood flow to the brain.

The effects of poor dental health on systemic diseases are well-documented, a matter that has led to a renewed interest in contribution of dental diseases to the systemic health outcomes. A report of the Surgeon General issued by United States Department of Health and Human Services (DHHS) about "Oral Health in America" identified the essential role that dental health plays in overall health and wellbeing. The report clearly indicated that the disparities in dental health status and access to dental care affected many of the United States people, and more specifically those with low income and members of racial/ethnic minority groups (National Institute of Dental and Craniofacial Research, 2000). Research have focused on the potential impact of oral diseases on systemic health such as cardiovascular disease (CVD), diabetes, respiratory diseases and adverse pregnancy outcomes (Dietrich & Garcia, 2005). Seymour *et al.* 2007) stated that dental diseases may represent a risk factor for systemic diseases, and hence controlling dental diseases is an essential approach in the prevention and management of these systemic diseases.

According to the Global Burden of disease study, stroke was the second largest cause of death globally, resulting in an annual mean estimate of 5.5 million deaths (Johnson *et al.*, 2019). Several epidemiologic studies have investigated the links between dental diseases and stroke. This link appears to be indirect or circumstantial, and the results from previous studies are inconsistent (Joshipura, 2002; Lin *et al.,* 2019; Sim *et al.,* 2008). The type of association between dental diseases and stroke has not been established. Joshipura (2002) reported that out of nine studies that evaluated tooth loss and periodontitis as risk factors for stroke, seven studies showed significant associations. Several studies claimed periodontitis as a risk factor for cerebral stroke in adults (Abolfazli *et al.*, 2011). Tooth loss, the ultimate end-result and remarkable indicator of periodontal disease, has been considered a risk factor for cerebral diseases and CVD (Lee *et al.*, 2019), and recent systematic reviews confirmed this association between tooth loss and stroke in adult patients (Cheng *et al.*, 2018; Fagundes *et al.,* 2020).

12.1. Oral Hygiene and Stroke

Stroke is an acute condition characterized by the sudden loss of blood supply to a region of the brain, causing injury to the cells and tissues. Stroke is typically divided into ischemic stroke and haemorrhagic stroke. Ischemic stroke, also known as cerebral ischemia, occurs when there is a blockage in the blood supply to a part of the brain. Haemorrhagic stroke occurs when a blood vessel supplying the brain ruptures and bleeds. Neurons begin to die within minutes of the onset of stroke because their oxygen supply is cut off. The brain damage caused by a stroke can impair a person's fundamental bodily functions such as movement, memory, and speech (Wood *et al*., 2022).

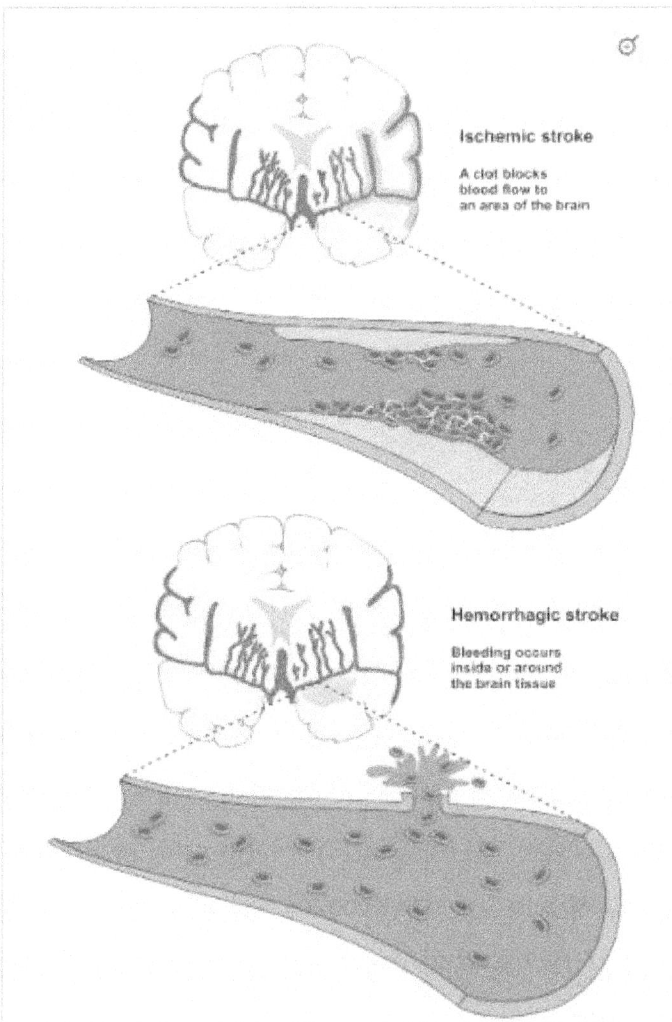

Difference between ischemic and haemorrhagic stroke

Bacterial infections can cause serious inflammatory reactions and spread to other mouth regions if not treated right at once. Other organs and tissues may experience significant alterations as a result of oral inflammation, which is not just limited to the oral cavity. It has been observed that hypertension, heart disease, diabetes, pulmonary lung disease (Hamamcilar *et al.,* 2018) and periodontal disease are all related to poor dental hygiene.

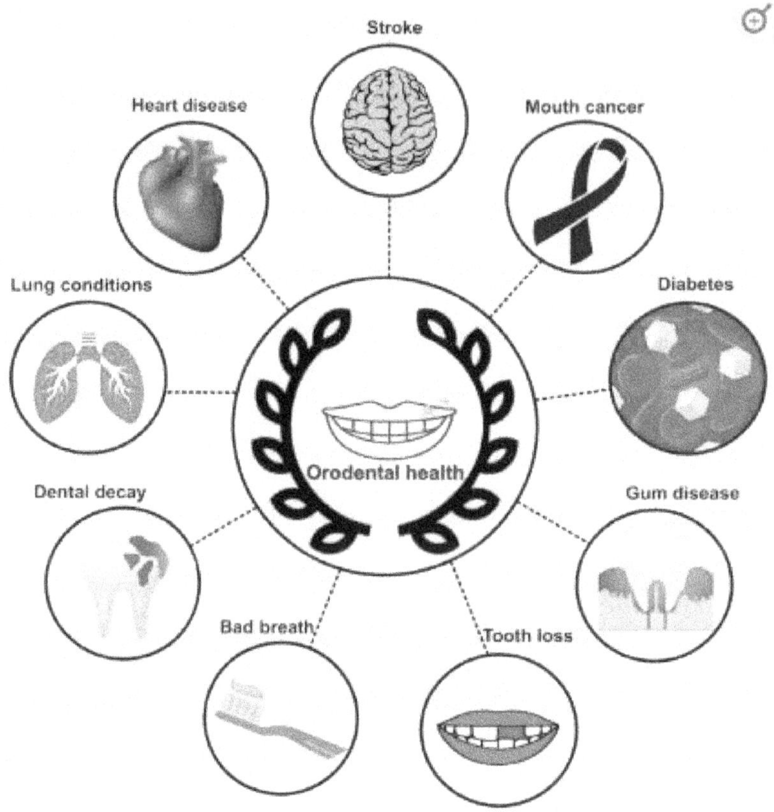

Link between oral health and general health

Oral bacteria can be sub-classified according to their oxygen requirements. The surface of soft tissues is an ideal site for the colonization of aerobic bacteria and fungi, where oxygen levels are high at these areas. As oxygen levels are less than 1%, anaerobic bacteria appear to predominate in the gingival sulcus and periodontal pocket (Ma *et al*., 2022). The species of oral bacteria vary considerably according to the stage of biofilm formation. Early colonizers found in the oral cavity are different species of streptococci and other natural microbiota, which have been not detected as respiratory bacterial pathogens (Aas *et al.,* 2005). In the later stages of colonization, biofilm microenvironment becomes anaerobic and ideal for more microbial species, such as *Tannerella forsythia*, *Treponema denticola*, *Fusobacterium nucleatum*, and *Porphyromonas gingivalis* to promote the risk of systemic infections. Some of these bacteria have been implicated in cerebrovascular diseases such as *Streptococcus mutans* involved in dental caries, *P. endodontalis* as a key pathogen in endodontic infections, and *P. gingivalis* involved in gingivitis and periodontitis. *Streptococcus* species are detectable in all atherosclerotic plaque samples. This mutant plays a critical role in accelerated onset of stroke in rats as well as in patients who have had a haemorrhagic stroke. The common and important viruses include cytomegalovirus, human papilloma virus, herpes simplex virus type 1 (HSV-1), and Epstein-Barr virus. Fungal infections in the oral environment are caused by Candida species, especially *Candida albicans*. In some cases, parasitic infections may also occur (Nakano *et al.*, 2011).

Oral hygiene indicators can elicit the incidence of stroke in various ways and to varying degrees depending on the stroke subtype. According to recent studies, ischemic stroke is more consistent with an infection theory, whereas haemorrhagic stroke is not often associated with dental or other infections and is significantly connected with hypertension (Gu *et al.,* 2022). Imaging investigations and physical examinations are frequently used to diagnose strokes. Studies on the prevention of stroke have begun to consider biomarkers, and several biomarkers have been identified (Dave *et al.*, 2022). Among them, it is commonly accepted that inflammatory biomarkers are associated with a higher risk of stroke aetiology and outcome (Xu *et al.,* 2022). In the post-stroke brain, damage signals and danger-associated molecular patterns are released by dying neuronal cells. Inflammatory cytokines are then released by activated microglia and peripheral leucocytes, which enhance the inflammatory response. Studies have reported that elevated inflammatory markers are associated with the risk of stroke recurrence and less favourable outcomes (Shi *et al.,* 2022). Several events such as reperfusion of tissue, oxidative stress, and microglial activity can promote cell death in the penumbra region, which can lead to secondary neuronal death and further increased damage to stroke area. These events can be triggered by a systemic inflammation, showing that the oro-dental diseases may aggravate the stroke condition (Alhadidi *et al.,* 2018). Through targeted modification of a single risk factor or a cluster of multiple risk factors at the individual and community level, stroke prevention programs have been designed to decrease the incidence of stroke in the last decade. There is much evidence about the association between stroke and oral health. However, the role of poor oral hygiene in the prevalence of stroke is controversial (Schmid *et al.,* 2010).

A new study presented at the American Stroke Association International Stroke Conference analysed the potential link between oral health and brain health among 40,000 adults without a history of stroke enrolled in the U.K. Biobank. Between 2014 and 2021, participants were screened for 105 genetic variants known to predispose people to have cavities, dentures, and missing teeth later in life. Signs of poor brain health, such as damage to the structure and white matter of the brain, were then screened via MRI images. (White matter is the large network of nerve fibres in your brain that allows the exchange of information and communication between different areas of your brain. It's called "white matter" because the nerve fibres are covered in a protective sheath called myelin, which gives the tissue its white colour.)

Researchers found, in their preliminary findings, that people who were genetically prone to cavities, missing teeth, or needing dentures had a higher amount of damage from a silent stroke, meaning a stroke that doesn't cause any noticeable symptoms, characterized by a 24% increase in the amount of white matter damage visible on the MRI images. Those with overall genetically poor oral health also had increased damage to the structure of the brain, characterized by a 43% change in structural damage visible on the MRI scans. After analysing the results, study explains, "Poor oral health may cause declines in brain health, so we need to be extra careful with our oral hygiene because it has implications far beyond the mouth." (Cyprien Rivier, Yale School of Medicine, American Heart Association).

12.2. Prevention Strategies

Brush twice a day for two minutes each time, and don't forget to clean tongue. Floss every day to remove plaque and bacteria from between teeth. Visit the dentist regularly for a dental check-up, cleaning, and screenings for oral cancers, periodontal/gum disease, caries, sleep apnea, and TMJ issues. Eat a healthy diet, with plenty of solid foods. Limit sugary drinks, including soda, concentrated juice, and carbonated water, or use a straw to limit contact with your teeth. Limit or avoid alcohol use. Avoid tobacco products, including smoking cigarettes and vaping. Use mouthwash to reduce plaque and bacteria. The person had a stroke, it's just as important to continue maintaining optimal oral hygiene to prevent any further complications. According to some studies reported, if a critically ill patient doesn't implement regular dental care following a stroke, they may develop ventilator-associated pneumonia. "An ounce of prevention is worth a pound of cure". In addition, if person have recently had a stroke, it's critically important that person follow a good oral care routine to protect overall health.

References

Aas J.A., Paster B.J., Stokes L.N., Olsen I., Dewhirst F.E. Defining the normal bacterial flora of the oral cavity. *J. Clin. Microbiol.* 2005; 43:5721–5732. doi: 10.1128/JCM.43.11.5721-5732.2005.

Abolfazli, N., Ghoreishizadeh, A., Ayramlu, H., Ghavimi, M., Ghoreishizadeh, M., & Salehsaber, F. (2011). Periodontal disease and risk of cerebral ischemic stroke. *Journal of Neurological Sciences*, 28(3), 307–316.

Cheng, F., Zhang, M., Wang, Q., Xu, H., Dong, X., Gao, Z., Chen, J. Wei, Y. , & Qin, F. (2018). Tooth loss and risk of cardiovascular disease and stroke: A dose-response meta-analysis of prospective cohort studies. *PLoS One*, 13, e0194563.

Cyprien Rivier, Yale School of Medicine, American Heart Association

Dave R.G., Geevar T., Aaron S., Ninan Benjamin R., Mammen J., Kumar S., Vijayan R., Gowri M., Nair S.C. Diagnostic utility of flow cytometry based coated-platelets assay as a biomarker to predict thrombotic or haemorrhagic phenotype in acute stroke. *Cytom. Part B Clin. Cytom.* 2022; 102:246–253. doi: 10.1002/cyto.b.22026.

Dietrich, T., & Garcia, R. I. (2005). Associations between periodontal disease and systemic disease: Evaluating the strength of the evidence. *Journal of Periodontology*, 76(Suppl 11S), 2175–2184.

Fagundes, N. C. F., Couto, R. S. D., Brandão, A. P. T., de Oliveira Lima, L. A. , de Oliveira Bittencourt, L. , de Souza-Rodrigues, R. D. Lima, R. R. (2020). Association between tooth loss and stroke: A systematic review. *Journal of Stroke and Cerebrovascular Diseases: The Official Journal of National Stroke Association*, 29, 104873.

Gu H.-Q., Yang K.-X., Lin J.-X., Jing J., Zhao X.-Q., Wang Y.-L., Liu L.-P., Meng X., Jiang Y., Li H. Association between high-sensitivity C-reactive protein, functional disability, and stroke recurrence in patients with acute ischaemic stroke: A mediation analysis. *EBioMedicine.* 2022; 80:104054. doi: 10.1016/j.ebiom.2022.104054.

Johnson CO, Nguyen M, Roth GA. Global, regional, and national burden of stroke, 1990–2016: a systematic analysis for the Global Burden of Disease Study 2016. Lancet Neurol. 2019; 18:439–458.

Joshipura, K. (2002). The relationship between oral conditions and ischemic stroke and peripheral vascular disease. *Journal of the American Dental Association*, 133(Suppl 1), 23s–30s.

Kim, H. D., Sim, S. J., Moon, J. Y., Hong, Y. C., & Han, D. H. (2010). Association between periodontitis and haemorrhagic stroke among Koreans: A case-control study. *Journal of Periodontology*, 81, 658–665.

Lin, H. W., Chen, C. M., Yeh, Y. C., Chen, Y. Y., Guo, R. Y., Lin, Y. P., & Li, Y. C. (2019). Dental treatment procedures for periodontal disease and the subsequent risk of ischaemic stroke: A retrospective population-based cohort study. *Journal of Clinical Periodontology*, 46, 642–649.

Ma K.S.K., Lai J.N., Veeravalli J.J., Chiu L.T., Van Dyke T.E., Wei J.C.C. Fibromyalgia and periodontitis: Bidirectional associations in population-based 15-year retrospective cohorts. *J. Periodontol.* 2022; 93:877–887. doi: 10.1002/JPER.21-0256.

Nakano K., Hokamura K., Taniguchi N., Wada K., Kudo C., Nomura R., Kojima A., Naka S., Muranaka Y., Thura M. The collagen-binding protein of *Streptococcus mutans* is involved in haemorrhagic stroke. *Nat. Commun.* 2011; 2:485. doi: 10.1038/ncomms1491.

National Institute of Dental and Craniofacial Research, 2000.

Seymour, Gregory. Good oral health is essential for good general health: The oral-systemic connection. Clinical Microbiology and Infection. 2007. 2(13). 10.1111/j.1469-0691.2007.01797. x.

Shi J., Yang Y., Yin N., Liu C., Zhao Y., Cheng H., Zhou T., Zhang Z., Zhang K. Engineering CXCL12 Biomimetic Decoy-Integrated Versatile Immunosuppressive Nanoparticle for

Ischemic Stroke Therapy with Management of Overactivated Brain Immune Microenvironment. *Small Methods.* 2022; 6:2101158. doi: 10.1002/smtd.202101158.

Woods JP, Heinecke EL, Luecke JW, Maldonado E, Ng JZ, Retallack DM, et al., editors. Pathogenesis of Histoplasma capsulatum. Semin Respir Infect; 2001.

HIGHLIGHTS

- During the menopausal, breastfeeding, and pregnant phases, dental care is considerably more important.
- Numerous studies have discovered evidence between poor oral health of the mother, the outcome of the pregnancy, and the offspring's dental health.
- Pregnant women should avoid eating too much sugar, brush their teeth frequently with fluoride toothpaste, and use fluoridated mouthwashes
- Effective care may be hampered by worries about early pregnancy treatments due to the risk of spontaneous abortion and early labor in later stages of pregnancy.
- Among a group of women (56%) who attended a dentist regularly either before or during their most recent pregnancy, dental caries was less common. A significant rise in dental caries (17.9%) was associated with preterm birth.

CHAPTER 13

Dental Health V/S Pregnancy

To sustain oral and dental health for a life time, effective and adequate care is essential. In women, dental care is much more important during pregnancy, breastfeeding, and menopausal periods. Pregnancy is not a disease state but instead it is a sign of being healthy. A healthy person is not expected to lose their teeth without any reason. The same rules are valid for pregnant women. If they take some simple precautions, they will not have any loss of teeth or other dental problems. Nevertheless, mothers are known to face tooth decay and gingival problems during pregnancy. Due to bad oral health in pregnancy, pregnant women can experience premature delivery, low birth weight baby, pre-eclampsia, gingival tissue ulcerations, pregnancy granuloma, gingivitis, pregnancy tumors (epulis gravidarum), loose teeth, mouth dryness, and dental erosions. The changing hormone levels in pregnancy directly affect gum problems, and indirectly, tooth decay (Dörtbudak *et al.*, 2005). The role of high levels of circulating estrogen is well established and associated with high prevalence of gingivitis and gingival hyperplasia. Progesterone in the serum is also seen to be associated with melasma, presenting a bilateral pigmentation or brown patches in the mid face region (Hemalatha *et al.*, 2013).

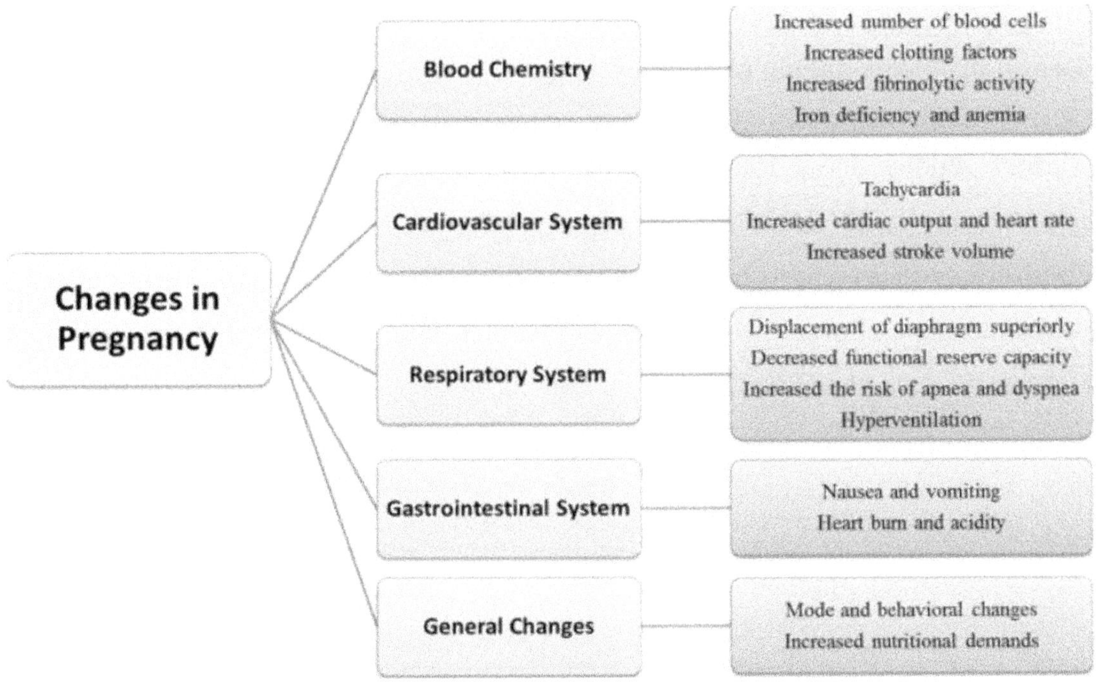

Key physiological change observed in various body systems during pregnancy

Pregnant women undergo hormonal balance changes during pregnancy. Many tissues undergo certain changes because the placenta produces higher levels of estrogen and progesterone during pregnancy. In this period, excessive sensitivity to irritations occurs in the gingiva. In pregnancy, gingivitis or epulis gravidarum, commonly known as pregnancy tumours, can be seen very often. Pregnancy gingivitis usually starts at the second month of gestation and reaches the highest level at the eighth month, and heals spontaneously after birth. They originate from pyogenic granuloma and disappear after 1-2 months. Surgical removal is recommended if they do not vanish spontaneously. Surgical excision can be performed by conventional methods or laser. Laser treatment may give more comfortable results to the patient because pyogenic granulomas have tendency to bleed. In fact, if they do not disturb the patient and if they do not bleed excessively, there is no need for treatment during pregnancy.

13.1. Dental problems during pregnancy

Various studies have found evidence linking together poor maternal oral health, pregnancy outcomes and dental health of the offspring. These may range from preterm delivery and low birth weight to higher risk of early caries among infants. Unfortunately, apart from self-maintenance of oral hygiene, pregnant women face several other barriers in achieving optimal oral health (Wood and Ito, 2000).

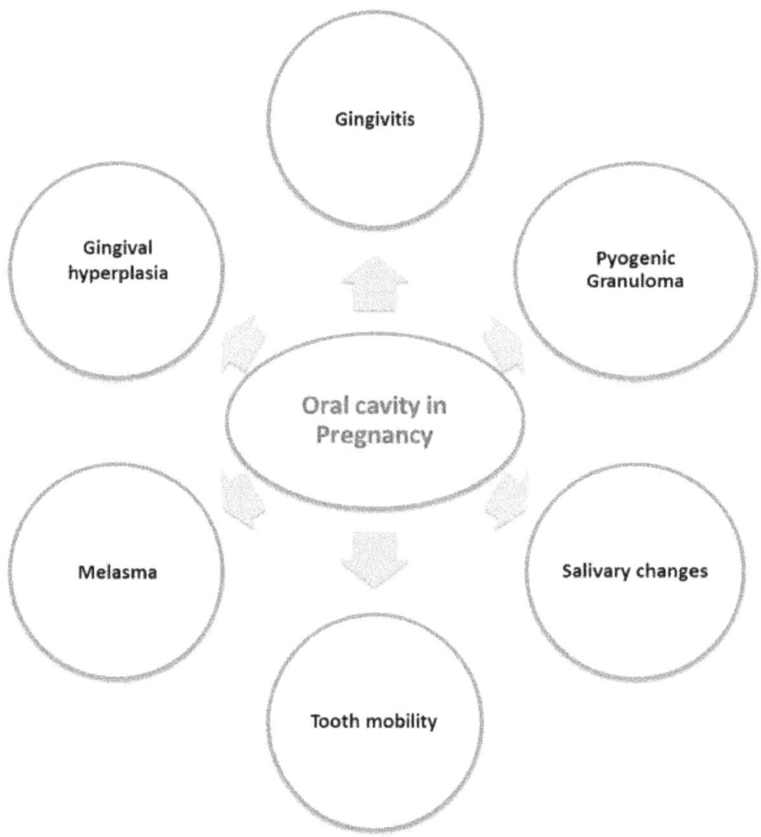

Oral health care measures adopted during pregnancy

13..1. Dental decay / caries: Pregnant women are more prone to tooth decay due to upturn in the acidic environment of oral cavity, increased consumption of sugary diet and carelessness toward oral health. Recurrent vomiting becomes common in pregnancy that enhances acidic environment leading to progress of carious pathogens and an increased demineralization making teeth prone to caries (Cheek and Gutsche 1993). Untreated carious lesions increase the incidence of abscess and cellulitis (Giglio *et al.,* 2009). It is advisable for pregnant women to limit sugary diet, brush regularly with fluoridated tooth paste and use over the counter fluoridated mouth rinses to counteract the effect of demineralization due to vomiting. The role of topical applications of fluoride is well accepted for the prevention of caries. Fluoride releasing restorative materials such as glass ionomers can inhibit secondary caries (Zafar, 2013). In addition, drugs such as methamphetamine that may further aggravate dental caries should be avoided (Amini and Casimassimo, 2010).

13.1.2. Periodontal disease: About 30% of pregnant women suffer from periodontal diseases. While the role of elevated levels of circulating estrogen is well established in higher prevalence of gingivitis and gingival hyperplasia during pregnancy, the association between pregnancy and oral diseases like periodontitis require further research. The role of elevated levels of inflammatory markers (i.e. interleukin 6, interleukin 8 and PGE2) has been found in the amniotic fluid of child bearing women having periodontal conditions, which is considered to be associated with premature labor and low birth weight (Huda *et al.,* 2015). Recent evidence clearly demonstrates that scaling and root planning is considered safe during pregnancy and improves both maternal and neonatal health (Michalowicz *et al.*, 2008). The management strategies to overcome periodontal disease in pregnant females embraces vigilant diagnosis by the dental health care professional, root planning/deep scaling and prescribing 0.12% daily chlorhexidine mouth rinses to limit the progress of disease. Chlorhexidine is categorized as FDA class B and measured safe to practice in pregnant women (Teratology Society Public Affairs Committee, 1994),

13.1.3. Gingivitis: Gingivitis or bleeding tender gums is the most common dental problem and contributes to around 60% –70% of pregnant women. Such conditions are common due to decreased immune response, hormonal fluctuations of estrogens and progesterone and changes in normal oral flora (RashidiMaybodi *et al.*, 2015). Commendations to improve the condition may comprise professional prophylaxis i.e. scaling, daily fluoridated tooth brushing, flossing and saline mouth rinses should be encouraged that may help in easing the irritant. In addition, chlorhexidine mouth rinses may provide added benefit (Bajaj, S. Tandon, 2011).

13.1.4. Tooth mobility : Due to hormonal rush mineral changes in lamina dura and disturbance in the periodontal ligament attachment, affect mobility of teeth leading to periodontal diseases

(Andrade *et al.*, 2004). This condition can be made reversible if given therapeutic doses of vitamin C along with removal of local gingival irritants (Rateitschak, 1967).

13.1.5. Tooth erosion: Tooth erosion, another unwanted dental problem is considered to be caused by pregnancy induced vomiting. It is understood that dental erosion can be effectively controlled with the use of a solution containing sodium bicarbonate that neutralizes the acid and prevents damages. It is advised to consult patient's physician and gastroenterologist to control the related medical conditions (Schroeder,1995).

13.2. Pharmacodynamics and pregnancy

Pregnancy is a phase having a high volume of drug distribution, decline in maximum plasma concentration, shorter plasma half-life, rise in lipid solubility and rate of clearance. Such dynamics contribute to an easy access of boundless drugs through the placenta, therefore compromising the health of the foetus (Schroeder *et al.*, 1995). Analgesics are used for a short or limited span of time to treat, cure and minimize the hassle of pain. Acetaminophen is the most common and safest analgesic used in pregnancy and is categorized in group B by the FDA classification (Grahame-Smith and Aronson 1992). Most antibiotics permitted by the dentist belongs to category B of FDA classification with exemption of gentamycin and doxycycline both of which fits in to class D. Metronidazole classified in group B is prohibited to be used in first trimester as the drug has teratogenic effects (Kazy *et al.,* 2005). Localized use of anaesthetics is considered safe when given properly and in precise dose. Anaesthetics such as lidocaine and prilocaine are categorized in class B whereas, mepivacaine, bupivacaine and epinephrine fits in class C of the FDA classification. Oral health care management of pregnant patients is considered to be a very important aspect. It is recommended to assess patient's current dental health status and then to educate her about the expected changes during pregnancy and measures that can be helpful to avoid pain and distress. The dental examination and treatment causes no harm to the fetus (during second and third trimester) in contrast to that if left untreated, e.g. dental decay may cause infant caries at a later stage. Similarly other procedures such as diagnosis, periodontal treatment, restorations and extractions are of no harm and are recommended to be performed during the middle trimester as organogenesis is complete by then (George *et al.*, 2010).

The first trimester is not considered to be an appropriate time for performing procedures. Organogenesis takes place during this period and is prone to risk of teratogens. Also, the risk of spontaneous abortions increases. In this trimester the organogenesis phase is complete and procedures such as emergent dento-alveolar and other electives procedures are safe to perform. Recommendations during this pace include: maintenance of oral hygiene and plaque control. It is appropriate to perform short dental procedures during the third trimester as there is not significant risk to the foetus. However, there is an increased risk of discomfort to the mother that can be reduced to a greater extent by proper positioning. Current evidence suggests that 'dental radiography' is measured as harmless in child bearing women. The safety directly rests upon the type and number of radiations to which the patients is exposed. A teratogen is defined as an agent that causes permanent alterations in the form or function of offspring upon exposure to the foetus. There is a wide range of medications that can lead to teratogenic effects and thus can be a reason to cause both functional and structural birth defects (Friedman, 1996).

Oral treatment during pregnancy is an important strategy to improve both maternal and infant oral health. However, dentists may be reluctant to provide dental treatment for a pregnant woman for a number of reasons, including concern about tetragenicity of various medications such as anaesthetics and antibiotics. Concerns about treatment in early pregnancy because of the possibility of spontaneous abortion and premature labour in later pregnancy may be barriers to effective care. A recent clinical trial by Michalowicz *et al.* (2008) found that providing dental treatment between 13- and 21-weeks' gestation was not associated with any adverse pregnancy outcomes. The treatment provided included scaling and root planting with local anaesthesia, and emergency dental treatment including restorative and surgical care. This supports work by Daniels *et al.* (2007), who found that dental care during pregnancy, including amalgam fillings, was not associated with birth outcomes or language development. This is somewhat in contrast to the precautionary recommendation from the National Health and Medical Research Council (NHMRC) (1999) that 'During pregnancy it is prudent to minimise exposure to all foreign substances including materials used in dental restorations. This indicates that placement or replacement of dental amalgam restorations should be avoided, especially during the first trimester'.

In one study, Hala Nadhim Kadhim of the University of Al-Watnia for Sciences & Technology in Iraq looked at the occurrence of dental caries in expectant mothers and how it related to their oral health and behavior. Twenty-eight (14%) of the 200 women who gave birth during the research period had dental caries. Sixteen ladies (6%) had treatment for dental caries among them. Mother's education and women in rural areas with more than three children showed a significant decrease in the frequency of dental caries. However, there is no connection between tobacco use or passive smoking and the development of dental caries. Compared to routine twice-daily brushing (6.8%), mothers who did not clean their teeth felt that the only reason they could lose a tooth due to dental caries was because they were pregnant (66.7%). Dental caries was less common in a group of women (56%) who saw a dentist on a regular basis either before or during their most recent pregnancy. A markedly increased rate of dental caries (17.9%) was linked to premature delivery.

13.3. Prevention of oral diseases in pregnancy

Standard preventive measures such as drinking of fluoridated water, twice daily use of fluoridated toothpaste and a low-sugar diet should be recommended for pregnant women (Griffin *et al.* 2007; Yeung, 2007). Fluoride supplements are not recommended in pregnancy as there is no evidence of effectiveness (ARCPOH 2006). A visit to the dentist is recommended for all pregnant women to check on periodontal conditions, as well as to minimise cariogenic oral flora through treatment of existing dental caries and advice on oral hygiene habits. Plaque control through meticulous oral hygiene is suggested for minimisation of gingivitis and to reduce the load of oral bacteria. Smoking cessation advice should be part of a preventive strategy for periodontal disease and for the range of conditions with which periodontal disease has been associated.

13.4. Oral issues of Newborn babies

13.4.1. Natal teeth, cysts: Occasionally, infants are born with tooth-like structures or develop them soon after birth (natal or neonatal teeth). These are usually in the mandible and are rare, occurring in 1 in 1,000 births (da Silva *et al.* 2008). Gingival cysts may also be present at birth and may occur in the midpalatal raphe (Epstein pearls), above the gum pads and especially in the maxilla (Bohn nodules), or on the alveolar crest (dental lamina cysts).

13.4.2. Prevention of transmission of Streptococcus mutans to the young baby: Early colonisation of the oral cavity with strep mutans bacteria has been associated with high rates of dental caries (Harris *et al.,* 2004; Law 2007). Reduction in maternal strep mutans through restorative and preventive regimens has been shown to reduce the caries levels in their young children (Ercan *et al.,* 2007). This risk can be further reduced with a low-sugar diet, good oral hygiene and appropriate fluoride exposure. However, parents should be advised to minimise the transfer of saliva from parent to child, and to ensure that their own oral care and oral health is as good as possible to reduce this risk factor in young children.

13.4.3. Use of dummies/pacifiers and finger sucking: There are general health benefits in the use of dummies, including analgesic effects, shorter hospital stays for pre-term babies and reduced risk of sudden infant death syndrome. However, prolonged use may have negative consequences such as dental malocclusion and otitis media (Sexton *et al.,* 2009). Non-nutritive sucking on a dummy, finger or thumb either very actively or for a long period can produce changes in the oral cavity. Duncan *et al.,* (2008) have found that dummy-sucking habits have a greater effect on the developing occlusion than that of a finger or thumb. However, a sucking habit with a dummy may be easier to break than with a finger or thumb. The majority of children.

References

Ajesh George, Maree Johnson, Anthony Blinkhorn, Sharon Ellis, Sameer Bhole and Shilpi Ajwani. Promoting oral health during pregnancy: current evidence and implications for Australian midwives. Journal of clinical nursing 19(23-24), 3324-3333,2010.

Amini H, Casimassimo PS. Prenatal dental care: a review. General Dentistry. 2010 May-Jun;58(3):176-180.

Bajaj, S. Tandon. The effect of Triphala and Chlorhexidine mouthwash on dental plaque, gingival inflammation, and microbial growth. Int J Ayurveda Res, 2 (2011), pp. 29-36.

da Silva CM, Ramos MM, Carrara CF, *et al.* Oral characteristics of newborns. Dental erosion and acid reflux disease. Ann Intern Med, 122 (1995), pp. 809-815.

Dörtbudak O, Eberhart R, Ulm M, Persson GR. Periododontitis, a Marker of Risk in Pregnacy for Preterm Birth. *J Clin Periodontol.* 2005; 32:45–52.

Duncan K, McNamara C, Ireland AJ, Sandy JR. Sucking habits in childhood and the effects on the primary dentition: findings of the Avon Longitudinal Study of Pregnancy and Childhood. *Int J Paediatr Dent.* 2008;**18**(3):178–188. doi: 10.1111/j.1365-263X.2007.00905. x.

Giglio, J.A, S.M. Lanni, D.M. Laskin, N.W. Giglio Oral health care for the pregnant patient . J Can Dent Assoc, 75 (2009), pp. 43-48.

Hemalatha V T, Hemalatha VT, Manigandan T, Sarumathi T, Aarthi Nisha V and Amudhan A. Dental considerations in pregnancy-a critical review on the oral care. J Clin Diagn Res. 2013 May;7(5):948-53.

James A. Giglio, Susan M. Lanni, Daniel M. Laskin, Nancy W. Giglio. JCDA. February 2009, Vol. 75, No. 1.43-48.

Kazy, Z, E. Puhó, A.E. Czeizel. Teratogenic potential of vaginal metronidazole treatment during pregnancy. Eur J Obstet Gynecol Reprod Biol, 123 (2005), pp. 174-178.

Klaus H. Rateitschak. Tooth mobility changes in pregnancy. Journal of periodontal research. Volume2, Issue3 June 1967, Pages 199-206

Neeti Bajaj and Shobha Tandon. The effect of Triphala and Chlorhexidine mouthwash on dental plaque, gingival inflammation, and microbial growth. Int J Ayurveda Res. 2011 Jan-Mar; 2(1): 29–36.

Patrick L. Schroeder, Steven J. Filler, Belinda Ramirez, David A. Lazarchik, Michael F. Vaezi, and Joel E. Richter. Dental Erosion and Acid Reflux Disease. 1 June 1995, Volume 122, Issue 11, Page: 809-815.

Rashidi Maybodi, F, A. Haerian Ardakani, F. Vaziri, A. Khabbazian, S. Mohammadi-Asl. CPITN changes during pregnancy and maternal demographic factors 'impact on periodontal health'. Iran J Reprod Med, 13 (2015), pp. 107-112.

Rateitschak. K.H. Tooth mobility changes in pregnancy. J Periodont Res, 2 (1967), pp. 199-206.

Schroeder, P.L, S.J. Filler, B. Ramirez, D.A. Lazarchik, M.F. Vaezi, J.E. Richter

Wood, A.J, S. Ito. Drug therapy for breast-feeding women. N Engl J Med, 343 (2000), pp. 118-126.

CHAPTER 14

Dental Caires V/S Diabetes mellitus

HIGHLIGHTS

- Diabetes is a chronic metabolic disease characterized by elevated blood sugar (glucose) levels.
- Although Type 1 and Type 2 diabetes mellitus can present similarly, clinical history and examination can differentiate them.
- Diabetes patients may be more susceptible to the development of dental cavities due to hyposalivation and increased salivary glucose levels.
- Mutans streptococci numbers and decreased salivary flow have been connected to diabetes mellitus metabolic control.
- By controlling your diabetes, lowering your blood sugar, visiting the dentist on a regular basis, brushing and flossing your teeth with fluoride toothpaste.

Diabetes is a long-term metabolic illness marked by high blood glucose (blood sugar) levels. Serious damage to the heart, blood vessels, eyes, kidneys, and nerves can result from diabetes over time. Hyper-glycemia is the primary clinical symptom of diabetes. Nevertheless, aberrant lipid and protein metabolism, as well as imbalances in minerals and electrolytes, are also linked to insulin shortage and/or insulin resistance. Type 1 diabetes mellitus, which is brought on by an absolute or nearly absolute insulin deficiency, and type 2 diabetes mellitus, which is typified by the presence of insulin resistance with an insufficient increase in insulin secretion to compensate, account for the vast majority of diabetic patients. Diabetes type 1 is a chronic illness in which the pancreas generates little or no insulin on its own. It was formerly referred to as juvenile diabetes or insulin-dependent diabetes. The most prevalent kind, type 2 diabetes, usually affects adults and is brought on by insufficient or resistant insulin production in the body. Type 2 diabetes has been far more common over the last three decades in all nations, regardless of wealth. Furthermore, diabetes that strikes a woman while she is pregnant is referred to as gestational diabetes. Lastly, there are numerous rare and varied forms of diabetes that result from genetic flaws, medications, infections, endocrinopathies, and pancreatic damage. These distinct and unrelated types of diabetes are included under "Other Specific Types."

Approximately 422 million individuals globally suffer from diabetes, with the majority residing in low- and middle-income nations. The disease is directly responsible for 1.5 million fatalities annually. Over the past few decades, there has been a steady rise in both the number of cases and the incidence of diabetes. India ranks second with 66.8 million people with diabetes in 2014 following China which ranks first with 96.2 million diabetics. International Diabetes Federation estimates that currently, more than 387 million people worldwide have diabetes and it is estimated to increase to 592 million by 2035. Several studies have reported a higher prevalence of caries for participants with Diabetes mellitus, particularly for those with poorly controlled Diabetes mellitus.

Diabetes around the world in 2021

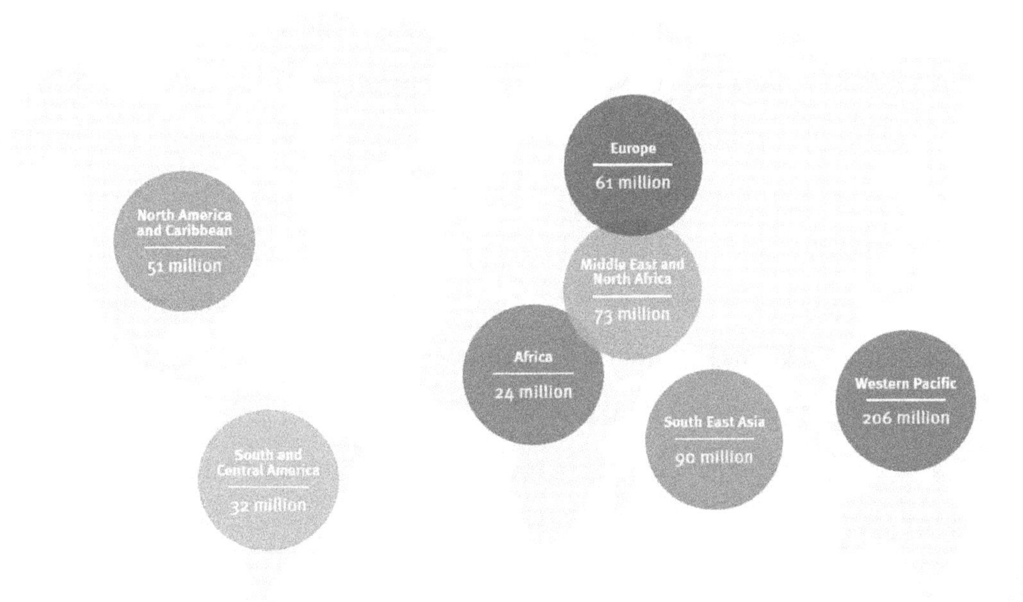

14.1. History and Physical condition

While Type 1 Diabetes mellitus and Type 2 Diabetes mellitus can present similarly, they can be distinguished based on clinical history and examination. Type 2 Diabetes mellitus patients are typically overweight/obese and present with signs of insulin resistance, including acanthosis nigricans, which are hyperpigmented, velvety patches on the skin of the neck, axillary, or inguinal folds. Patients with a longer course of hyperglycemia may have blurry vision, frequent yeast infections, numbness, or neuropathic pain. The clinicians must ask the patient bout any recent skin changes in their feet during each visit. The diabetic foot exam, including the monofilament test, should be a part of the routine physical exam (Amit Sapra and Priyanka Bhandari, 2023). According to the American Diabetes Association (ADA), a diagnosis of diabetes is through any of the following: An HbA1c level of 6.5% or higher; A fasting plasma glucose level of 126 mg/dL (7.0 mmol/L) or higher (no caloric intake for at least 8 hours); A two-hour plasma glucose level of 11.1 mmol/L or 200 mg/dL or higher during a 75-g OGTT; A random plasma glucose of 11.1 mmol/L or 200 mg/dL or higher in a patient with symptoms of hyperglycemia (polyuria, polydipsia, polyphagia, weight loss) or hyperglycemic crisis (American Diabetes Association, 2010). The ADA recommends screening adults aged 45 years and older regardless of risk, while the United States Preventative Service Task Force suggests screening individuals between 40 to 70 years who are overweight (Selph *et al.,* 2008).

14.2. Relationship between Dental Caries and Diabetes mellitus

The oral cavity structure can be affected by diabetes, which may result in several complications including dental caries, periodontal disease, oral mucosal diseases, and saliva dysfunction that have a significant effect on the quality of life of diabetic patients. Also, untreated oral diseases may increase the risk of poor metabolic control (Leite *et al.,* 2013). The relationship between diabetes and dental caries has received the attention of researchers because both of the diseases are associated with carbohydrates. The insulin deficiency in diabetes may lead to hyposalivation and elevated salivary glucose levels, which may put diabetic patients at a high risk of caries development (Malvania, *et al*., 2016). Saliva composition is an important factor in determining the prevalence of caries and oral health. It maintains the integrity of oral tissues, provides protection against immunologic bacterial, fungal, and viral infections (Bretas *et al.*, 2008) and controls the equilibrium between demineralization and remineralization in a cariogenic environment. Also, salivary buffers can stabilize pH in plaque, thus preventing demineralization of enamel (Animireddy *et al.,* 2014). Patients with diabetes have been reported to complain of dry mouth and salivary dysfunction leading to a reduction of salivary flow rate, lower buffer capacity, increased risk for dental caries, and bacterial infections (Al-Maskari*, et al.*, 2011).

Increasing the level of glucose in saliva affects the activity of microorganisms. *Streptococcus mutans* and *Lactobacillus* are considered to be related to caries and are the most cariogenic bacteria because they have the ability to create a low pH environment and progression of caries (Chase *et al.,* 2004). Research studies show that *Streptococcus mutans* and *Lactobacillus* found in stimulated saliva explain better the development of caries than *Streptococcus mutans* and *Lactobacillus* found in plaque. For this reason, the combined analysis of dental caries, salivary components, and bacterial pathogens in saliva is a powerful method of following the oral diseases in children with type 1 diabetes mellitus (Mohamed *et al.*, 2016).

The main complications of Diabetes mellitus affect the organs and tissues rich in capillary vessels, such as the kidney, retina and nerves. These complications are secondary to the development of microangiopathy (Hanssen, 1997). Similar changes in small vessels can be found in the oral tissues. Oral complications include dental caries, periodontal disease, and tooth mobility that is influenced by saliva. (Frantzis *et al.*, 1971). Diabetic patients are associated with intensive loss of fluid due to polyuria, reduced response to infections, impaired connective tissue metabolism, and various microvascular changes. These factors are responsible for various oral diseases in diabetic patients including xerostomia, salivary gland dysfunction, increased susceptibility to bacterial, viral and fungal infection, periapical abscesses, loss of teeth, taste impairment, lichen planus, burning mouth syndrome, and altered orthodontic tooth movements (Listgarten *et al.*, 1974). A very high and appalling prevalence of dental caries is found in diabetic patients compared to nondiabetics. It has been reported in the literature from previous studies that risk of dental caries is more prevalent in patients with type-II Diabetes mellitus compared to nondiabetics. Diabetes mellitus is responsible for causing ascendancy in the proportion and activity of saliva that impacts the oral health.

14.3. Prevalence of dental caries in children with type 1 diabetes

Type 1 diabetes mellitus is a chronic autoimmune disease characterized by the destruction of pancreatic beta cells and insulin deficiency, and affects over half a million children worldwide (Novotna *et al.*, 2015). Numerous epidemiological studies have reported that type 1 diabetes increases the risk for cardiovascular diseases, kidney disease and cognitive decline in children and adolescents (Tonoli *et al.*, 2014). Additionally, a growing number of studies indicate an underlying link between type 1 diabetes and oral complications, including periodontal diseases and dental caries (Miko *et al.,* 2010). Dental caries is the most common chronic infectious disease, and has posed an international public health challenge, especially in young children (Colak *et al.*, 2013). Screening and preventive treatment are necessary to avoid dental caries before they become incurable in the high-risk population. However, the exact prevalence of dental caries remains controversial in children and adolescents with type 1 diabetes, especially in those with poor metabolic control (Carneiro *et al.*, 2015). Moreover, several studies have showed that a higher prevalence was observed in diabetic adolescents with poor metabolic control compared to patients with good metabolic control (Lai *et al.,* 2017). Since parents are the primary caregivers for their children's oral health, their role is crucial in terms of oral health. According to research, parents of children with diabetes frequently take little notice of their child's untreated dental cavities and fail to recognize the connection between oral health and diabetes.

As of right now, there is no conclusive proof between diabetes mellitus with dental caries. The majority of previously published clinical trials were small, cross-sectional in design, and the outcomes were not very conclusive. Some studies found that patients with diabetes had higher levels of decaying, missing, or filled surfaces or teeth (DMFS or DMFT index) or its components than people without diabetes, whereas other studies found no discernible changes. Furthermore, the question of whether blood sugar regulation affects dental caries has only been somewhat investigated, with sporadic promising results in tiny clinical trials. People with uncontrolled diabetes had a significantly greater prevalence of untreated caries than people with metabolically sound conditions, according to the population-based Korean National Health and Nutrition Examination Survey. The majority of these clinical studies linking diabetes to dental caries, however, were of low quality, highly susceptible to bias, and had total sample sizes of fewer than 300 participants, indicating that the majority of the studies may have been underpowered. Thus, to raise the evidence grade, carefully planned, extensive clinical and epidemiological investigations are required.

14.4. Prevention and Control

Maintaining proper oral hygiene is crucial for overall health and wellbeing—it even has an impact on our sense of self. Additionally, it aids in preventing gum and tooth disease-related discomfort and infections as well as pain and infections from these conditions. It is much more crucial to take care of your teeth if you have diabetes. Treatment for gum disease has the potential to decrease white blood cells and eventually help lower blood sugar. These are the primary means by which the body combats oral infections. Making regular dentist appointments is essential to preventing problems. Brush teeth at least twice a day using fluoride toothpaste. Floss teeth at least once a day. Tell to dentist that person have diabetes issues. Consult a dentist if your gums are red, inflamed, or bleed easily. These might be signs of gum disease. Other symptoms include loose teeth, mouth pain, or dry mouth. Avoid smoking as it can worsen diabetes and increase the risk of gum disease.

References

Al-Maskari A. Y., Al-Maskari M. Y., Al-Sudairy S. Oral manifestations and complications of diabetes mellitus: a review. *Sultan Qaboos University Medical Journal.* 2011;11(2):179–186.

American Diabetes Association. Diagnosis and classification of diabetes mellitus. Diabetes Care. 2010 Jan;33 Suppl 1: S62-9.

Animireddy D., Reddy Bekkem V. T., Vallala P., Kotha S. B., Ankireddy S., Mohammad N. Evaluation of pH, buffering capacity, viscosity and flow rate levels of saliva in caries-free, minimal caries and nursing caries children: an in vivo study. *Contemporary Clinical Dentistry.* 2014;5(3):324–328. doi: 10.4103/0976-237x.137931.

Bretas L. P., Rocha M. E., Vieira M. S., Rodríguez A. Flow rate and buffering capacity of the saliva as indicators of the susceptibility to caries disease. *Pesquisa Brasileira em Odontopediatria e Clínica Integrada.* 2008;8(3):289–293.

Chase I., Berkowitz R. J., Mundorff-Shrestha S. A., Proskin H. M., Weinstein P., Billings R. Clinical outcomes for Early Childhood Caries (ECC): the influence of salivary mutans streptococci levels. *European Journal of Dentistry.* 2004;5(3):143–146.

Lai S., Cagetti M. G., Cocco F., et al. Evaluation of the difference in caries experience in diabetic and non-diabetic children-a case control study. *PLoS One.* 2017;12(11) doi: 10.1371/journal.pone. 0188451.e01884510188451.

Leite R. S., Marlow N. M., Fernandes J. K. Oral Health and type 2 diabetes. *American Journal of the Medical Sciences.* 2013;345(4):271–273. doi: 10.1097/maj.0b013e31828bdedf.

Malvania E. A., Sheth S. A., Sharma A. S., Mansuri S., Shaikh F., Sahani S. Dental caries prevalence among type II diabetic and nondiabetic adults attending a hospital. *Journal of International Society of Preventive and Community Dentistry.* 2016;6(9):232–236. doi: 10.4103/2231-0762.197202.

Miko S, Ambrus SJ, Sahafian S, Dinya E, Tamas G, Albrecht MG. Dental caries and adolescents with type 1 diabetes. Br Dent J 2010; 208(6):12. doi: 10.1038/sj.bdj.2010.290.

Mohamed H. G., Idris S. B., Mustafa M., et al. Influence of type 2 diabetes on prevalence of key periodontal pathogens, salivary matrix metalloproteinases, and bone remodeling markers in sudanese adults with and without chronic periodontitis. *International Journal of Dentistry.* 2016; 2016:9. doi: 10.1155/2016/6296854.6296854.

Selph S, Dana T, Blazina I, Bougatsos C, Patel H, Chou R. Screening for type 2 diabetes mellitus: a systematic review for the U.S. Preventive Services Task Force. Ann Intern Med. (2015) 162:765–76. doi: 10.7326/M14-2221.

CHAPTER

15

Use of Antibiotics in Dentistry

HIGHLIGHTS

- Current guidelines state that antibiotics should only be used following the eradication of the infecting agents.
- One of the earliest antiseptic agents to be suggested for use against dental caries was chlorhexidine, and it has shown out to be the most successful.
- Children who have dental infections are treated with antibiotics by dentists to lower their risk of bacteraemia; however, antibiotic therapy should not be used as a substitute for removing the source of the illness.
- In the field of dentistry, antimicrobial treatments that are often administered and deemed safe during pregnancy
- When antibiotics are used often and on a regular basis to treat dental infections, resistant bacteria, including multidrug-resistant pathogens, frequently emerge.

Antibiotic medicines, endodontic therapy, and surgical procedures could all be used to treat dental infections. To stop more damage, the infected tooth should be surgically managed as soon as possible. In severe situations, this may involve debridement, irrigation, and incision and drainage (I&D). Additionally, it is advised to administer intravenous antibiotics based on bacterial cultures and sensitivity in patients exhibiting evidence of systemic involvement. According to current recommendations, antibiotics ought to be used only after the infectious sources have been eradicated. Following surgical treatments, they should be recommended for two to three days in a row. Extended periods of antibiotic treatment did not yield noteworthy advantages and are not advised. Shortly after the introduction of penicillin and, in later years, vancomycin, the notion that dental caries could be treated by antibiotics was tested in laboratory animals. This idea was not pursued, mainly because of the growing fear that pathogenic bacteria may become tolerant to the regular use of sublethal doses of antibiotic. Interestingly, and supportive of the bacterial cause of dental caries, children receiving regular doses of antibiotics for amelioration of symptoms associated with cystic fibrosis exhibited significantly less tooth decay compared with the nonmedicated population. Chlorhexidine was one of the first antiseptic agents proposed for use against dental caries and has proved to be the most effective. (Kohler and Andreen, 1994; Wright *et al.,* 1992).

15.1. Indications of Antibiotics

Antibiotics are suggested in the cases of prophylaxis for local and focal infections, besides, for the treatment of odontogenic and nonodontogenic infections (Poveda Roda et al., 2007). Antibiotics are not indicated for all odontogenic infections; they should not be used instead of removal of the source of infections. In the case of infection, I&D, debridement, and endodontic management followed by systemic antibiotic therapy are recommended. Moreover, the practitioners should also bear in mind that the antibiotic prophylaxis is indicated in a few specified conditions (Schwartz and Larson, 2007). Antibiotic prophylaxis is a necessary option in cases of immunosuppressed patients, patients with a history of cancer, individuals with infective endocarditis, patients with metabolic disorders (such as diabetes and splenectomies), patients with prosthetic joints, in-dwelling catheters, neurosurgical shunts, valvular heart diseases, surgical pulmonary shunts, hypertrophic cardiomyopathy, mitral valve prolapsed, and prosthetic heart valves. In susceptible patients, some procedures enhance the risk of infection such as dental extraction, surgical periodontal procedures, dental implant placement, reimplantation of teeth, endodontic procedures or endodontics surgeries, subgingival placement of antibiotic fibers or strips, and intra-ligamentary local anaesthetic injections (Tong *et al.,* 2000). Prophylaxis for healthy patients is also suggested in special dental practices, such as surgery for benign tumors, bone grafting, implant placement, periapical surgery, and removal of impacted teeth (Kumar et al., 2014).

15.2. Antibiotic Advice for Childrens

Anatomical and physiological differences between children and adults such as the amount of their body water and fat, the maturation of the immune system, the volume of protein, and the level of liver enzymes should be considered while prescribing antibiotics for children (Caviglia *et al.,* 2014). Dentists treat children with antibiotics to reduce the risk of bacteraemia caused by dental infections; however, antibiotic therapy should not be used as an alternative method for elimination of an infection source (Cherry *et al.,* 2012). Furthermore, antibiotic resistance owing to inappropriate use, prescribing antibiotics in the wrong situation and for a too long period in children is a global concern. Therefore, dental practitioners should be aware of proper antibiotic choices and indications of antibiotic therapy for children under 13 years (Peedikayil 2011).

15.3. Antibiotic advice during the pregnancy

The drug prescription during the pregnancy should be done more cautiously, as the inappropriate prescription could irrecoverably harm the foetus. In dental practice, the main agents that are commonly used during pregnancy and are considered to be safe during this period are analgesics, anesthetic agents, and antibiotics. Food and Drug Administration (FDA) has classified drugs into 5 groups (A, B, C, D, and X) based on their risk factors during pregnancy and most of the antibiotics are classified to be in class B of FDA arrangement. Furthermore, the pregnant patients should receive a complete adult dose with the usual length of treatment (Donaldson and Goodchild, 2012). The physiological changes of pregnancy can affect the condition of the oral cavity such as increasing the risk of (In detail chapter – 13) dental infections. (Kloetzel *et al.,* 2011).

15.4. Common Prescribed Antibiotics in Dentistry

The first antibiotics were used to treat patients in the middle of the 20th century. These included medications that contained sulfa and those made from natural chemicals produced by microorganisms, including the 1941 discovery of penicillin. Antibiotics have subsequently been utilized in clinical and pharmaceutical research to address the problems caused by bacterial infections. Systemic antibiotics demonstrated potential usefulness early in the prevention or treatment of dental caries. Beta-lactam antibiotics are the antimicrobial agents that contain beta-lactam ring in their molecular structure (this ring includes a three-carbon and one-nitrogen cyclic amine structure). This group of antibiotics is bactericidal agents that act against many Gram-positive, Gram-negative, and anaerobic bacteria via inhibiting the synthesis of the cell wall. Beta-lactam antibiotics are categorized into five classes: Penicillin, Cephalosporins, Penems, Carbapenems, and Monobactams (Kloos *et al.*, 1991). The following antibiotics are generally prescribed for treatment of dental infections (Table- 3).

Table-3 -Commonly used antibiotics in Dentistry

Antibiotic	Mode of Action	Category	Side effects
Penicillin	Inhibit the synthesis of the peptidoglycan layer of the bacterial cell walls	Gram-positive *Streptococci* and *Staphylococci*, as well as some gram-negative bacteria	Diarrhoea, hypersensitivity, nausea, rash, neurotoxicity, and urticaria
Tetracyclines	Inhibit protein synthesis by binding to the 30S ribosomal subunit in the mRNA translation complex	Broad-spectrum antibiotics	Cramps or burning of the stomach, diarrhoea, sore mouth or tongue, skin photosensitivity, headache rarely, and vision problems, with damage to the kidneys also having been reported
Metronidazole	Inhibit nucleic acid synthesis when it is reduced by disrupting DNA	Bactericidal action against oral obligate anaerobes	Nausea, a metallic taste, headaches, flushing of the skin, tachycardia, loss of appetite, and shortness of breath, have been reported
Macrolides	Inhibit ribosomal translation by reversibly binding to the P site on the 50S subunit of the bacterial ribosome	Beta-haemolytic *streptococci*, *pneumococci*, *staphylococci*, and *enterococci*, having a slightly wider antimicrobial spectrum than penicillin	Myopathy, long QT syndrome, enterohepatic recycling, and cholestasis
Clindamycin	Inhibitor of bacterial protein synthesis by disrupting ribosomal translocation	Treat anaerobic infections caused by susceptible anaerobic bacteria, including dental, respiratory tract, skin, soft tissue, and peritonitis infections as well as penicillin-resistant infections.	Diarrhoea, pseudomembranous colitis, nausea, vomiting, abdominal pain or cramps, and contact dermatitis

15.5. Antimicrobial agents against oral pathogens

The application of systemic antibiotics has gradually reduced during recent decades, with other antimicrobial agents having been developed to target oral bacteria that cause oral diseases, such as fluoride, chlorhexidine, quaternary ammonium salts, and antimicrobial peptides (AMPs) (Table -4).

Table- 4- Antimicrobial agents used in Dentistry

Agent	Mode of Action	Active against	Forms available
Fluoride	Inhibition of enolase results in the growth inhibition and reduced acid production of oral streptococci, such as *S. mutans*	Antibacterial agent	Supplemented in small quantities to drinking water or, products such as mouthwashes, toothpastes, and oral supplements
Chlorhexidine	Damaging the inner cytoplasmic membrane. "gold standard" of antiplaque agents	Gram-positive and gram-negative bacteria, facultative anaerobes, aerobes, and yeasts.	Rinsing Solutions
Quaternary ammonium salts	Quaternary amines bind to the negatively charged bacteria cells to disturb the electric balance and can also promote the bacterial lysis by binding to bacterial membranes	Antimicrobial agents, surfactants, fabric softeners, and antistatic agents	Rinsing Solutions
Antimicrobial peptides	Cell permeabilization followed by membrane disruption, which depends on their relatively strong electrostatic attraction to negatively charged bacterial cells	Antimicrobial activities against a broad spectrum of microorganisms	Rinsing Solutions

Remineralizing Agents	Natural repair mechanism of teeth to restore the presence of minerals to the hydroxyapatite	Clinically to treat dental caries	Calcium phosphate nanoparticles, polydopamine, oligopeptides, theobromine, and arginine

15.6. Antimicrobial resistance

Antimicrobial resistance is a grave public health and patient care issue. Antimicrobial resistant infections are exceedingly problematic in regards to the treatment of infectious diseases. Consequently, prudent use of antimicrobials demands the highest priority to prevent antimicrobial resistance, ensure patient safety and improve healthcare. Multiple studies reported that dental surgeons frequently prescribed inappropriate antibiotics which ultimately promote antimicrobial resistance (Cope and Chestnutt, 2014). Currently enormous amounts of antibiotics are prescribed and consumed because of dental infective disorders around the planet. Regular and frequent use of antibiotics in dental infection often causes long-term public health troubles by leading to the development of resistant microbes including multidrug-resistant pathogens. This may be all the more tragic if there was minimal benefit to patient care by giving the antibiotic in these circumstances (Lee *et al.*, 2013).

The formation of microbial biofilms, such as dental plaque, is an important reason for the failure of antimicrobial therapy and the promotion of antibiotic resistance. However, the molecular mechanisms underlying the survival of biofilm cells are still not completely understood. There are three potential reasons for this issue: the first is biofilm-specific protection against oxidative stress; the second concerns the biofilm-specific expression of efflux pumps to pump out antibiotics; and the third is protection provided by matrix polysaccharides that can reduce the diffusion of antibiotics, which may play a significant role in antibiotic resistance. These mechanisms are associated with both bacterial and fungal biofilms and are often surprisingly similar between distantly related organisms (Li, *et al.,* 2011). Apart from these mechanisms, recent studies have shown that fluoride-resistant microorganisms, which are relatively different from fluoride-sensitive ones in growth and metabolic activity, may be another key factor in antibiotic resistance. The fluoride-resistant microorganisms can be detected in xerostomia patients who have been treated with a much higher concentration of fluoride. Therefore, the existence of fluoride-resistant microorganisms, especially fluoride-resistant *S. mutans*, will influence the effects of caries prevention and treatment and even lead to the failure of caries management. Furthermore, the common treatment (antibiotics or antimicrobial agent treatment) cannot completely inhibit the growth and metabolic activity of bacteria. Oral microorganisms left in cavities not only can induce the recurrence of dental caries but also do harm the pulp system, particularly when cariogenic bacteria, such as *S. mutans*, are the dominant microorganisms in dental plaque (Hayati *et al.,* 2011).

Incision, drainage, and pulp debridement are examples of surgical procedures that require antibiotic medication to control dental infections. To treat tooth infections, dentists prefer to recommend co-amoxiclav or amoxicillin and metronidazole. Clindamycin is an additional medication for individuals who are allergic to penicillins. The likelihood of prescribing the wrong antibiotic is decreased by precise knowledge of oral bacteria, the nature of oral diseases, and the pharmacokinetics of antibiotics. These antibiotics are never used clinically because of many adverse effects such as hypersensitivity reactions, supra infections and teeth staining. A high concentration of antibiotics causes coagulation of the intracellular constituents. As a result, the cytoplasm becomes congealed, with a resulting reduction in leakage. Many investigations are being conducted to prevent or minimize the use of antibiotics in order to lessen their unfavourable side effects.

References

Caviglia I., Techera A., García G. Antimicrobial therapies for odontogenic infections in children and adolescents. Literature review and clinical recomendations. *Journal Oral of Research.* 2013;3(1):50–56. doi: 10.17126/joralres.2014.013.

Cherry W. R., Lee J. Y., Shugars D. A., White R. P., Jr, Vann W. F., Jr Antibiotic use for treating dental infections in children. *The Journal of the American Dental Association.* 2012;143(1):31–38. doi: 10.14219/jada.archive.2012.0015.

Hayati. F, A. Okada, Y. Kitasako, J. Tagami, and K. Matin, "An artificial biofilm induced secondary caries model for in vitro studies," *Australian Dental Journal*, vol. 56, no. 1, pp. 40–47, 2011.

Kohler B., Andreen I., Jonsson B. (1984). The effect of caries-preventive measures in mothers on dental caries and the oral presence of the bacteria Streptococcus mutans and lactobacilli in their mothers. *Arch Oral Biol* 29:879-883.

Kumar A., Singh M., Gupta A. Prophylactic use of antibiotics in dentistry–a review. 2014.

Li, X., V. Alvarez, W. J. Harper, and H. H. Wang, "Persistent, toxin-antitoxin system-independent, tetracycline resistance-encoding plasmid from a dairy *Enterococcus faecium* isolate," *Applied and Environmental Microbiology*, vol. 77, pp. 7096–7103, 2011.

M. Donaldson and J. H. Goodchild, "Is clindamycin dangerous?" *General Dentistry*, vol. 65, pp. 12–15, 2017.

Schwartz A.B., Larson E.L. Antibiotic prophylaxis and postoperative complications after tooth extraction and implant placement: A review of the literature. *J. Dent.* 2007;35:881–888. doi: 10.1016/j.jdent.2007.08.003.

Tong D. C., Rothwell B. R. Antibiotic prophylaxis in dentistry: a review and practice recommendations. *The Journal of the American Dental Association.* 2000;131(3):366–374. doi: 10.14219/jada.archive.2000.0181.

Tong, Z, L. Zhou, W. Jiang et al., "An in vitro synergetic evaluation of the use of nisin and sodium fluoride or chlorhexidine against *Streptococcus mutans*," *Peptides*, vol. 32, no. 10, pp. 2021–2026, 2011.

Wright JT, Cutter GR, Dasanayake AP, Stiles HM, Caufield PW. 1992. Effect of conventional dental restorative treatment on bacteria in saliva. *Community Dent Oral Epidemiol*. 20(3):138–143.

CHAPTER

16

Vaccine Approach

HIGHLIGHTS

- Antibiotics are frequently used to treat dental caries, with the goal of eliminating or inhibiting biofilm formation in the oral cavity.
- An antibody, commonly referred to as an immunoglobulin (Ig), is a big Y-shaped protein that is made by plasma cells and is used to neutralize foreign substances like viruses and bacteria.
- Procedures where the animals must be kept as antibody producers for an extended length of time or that call for the synthesis of significant quantities of polyclonal antibodies.
- When it comes to animal welfare, using laying hens to produce antibodies is a refinement and a decrease in the use of animals.
- Generally speaking, chickens have a similar immune response to mammals and are strong makers of antibodies.

Oral and Dental Health have improved enormously over the last century in the urbanized countries, but the prevalence of dental caries in the developing countries like India remains a considerable clinical problem. At present various caries defensive strategies are in use like oral health education, chemical and mechanical control of plaque, use of fluorides, application of pit and fissure sealants etc. A lot of these approaches can be broadly effective, profitable. However behavioural or cultural barriers to their use encompass constant the epidemic of dental disease in the mouths of many people on a global level. Antibiotics are constantly in use for treating dental caries, it has been used in aspire of eradication or inhibition of biofilm in the oral cavity (in detail chapter – 15). Due to the over usage and side effects of antibiotics new approach for combating dental caries is through the development of an efficient vaccine that is well suited for public health applications especially in environments that do not lend themselves to regular health care.

16.1. Prevention of Dental caries - Vaccine approaches

Vaccine approaches for eliciting an IgA or IgG response are being debated. Results using animal models have been promising, especially coupled with newer forms of antigen delivery, such as liposomes, but safety and efficacy in humans have not yet been demonstrated. Whether mutans streptococci alone are the appropriate target, or if other bacteria must be included, is still an open question. Moreover, targeting members of the indigenous flora, as opposed to exogenous pathogens, requires that immunoglobulins distinguish self from non-self-antigens so as not to induce an autoimmune reaction. Despite some difficulties that must be overcome, the development of an inexpensive and effective vaccine would be a tremendous tool for combating dental caries, especially in developing countries (Michalek and Childers, 1990; Smith and Taubmar, 1995).

An antibody also known as an immunoglobulin (Ig), is a large Y-shape protein produced by plasma cells that is used by the immune system to identify and neutralize foreign objects such as bacteria and viruses. Antibodies can occur in two physical forms, a soluble form that is secreted from the cell, and a membrane-bound form that is attached to the surface of a B cell and is referred to as the B cell receptor (BCR). In humans, five classes of immunoglobulins, also called isotypes (IgG, IgM, IgA, IgD and IgE), differ in their physicochemical and serological properties, and in the amino acid sequence of their constant regions. In their monomeric form, all classes exhibit the same basic structure: two heavy (H) and two light (L) chains. While IgG, IgD and IgE consist of a single monomeric unit, the IgM and IgA classes are composed of monomers that associate to form pentamers and dimers, respectively. Formation of these polymers requires an additional polypeptide chain termed the J chain. Serological analysis of immunoglobulins of the same class revealed the existence of additional heterogeneity and resulted in the subdivision of classes into subclasses. In addition to the five major classes, there are four subclasses of IgG in humans (IgG1 to IgG4) and in mice (IgG1, IgG2a, IgG2b and IgG3), and two subclasses of IgA in humans (IgA1 and IgA2).

16.2. Generation of antibodies

The immunisation of laboratory animals to induce a humoral and or cellular immune response is a routine procedure performed worldwide (Marlies Leenaars, 1999). The selection of the animal species for the production of polyclonal antibodies depends on the amount of antiserum needed and the ease of obtaining blood samples. Polyclonal antibodies (antisera) are commonly produced by injection of the immunogen (antigen) of interest in to an animal, often in combination with an adjuvant to increase the immune response. The antibody response can be enhanced by subsequent booster injections of the antigen with or without adjuvant. Blood samples are obtained from the animal to assess the level of antibodies produced, and once a sufficiently high titre has been reached, the antiserum is prepared by blood collection followed by serum preparation, with subsequent purification of antibodies from the serum is required. For protocols requiring the production of large volumes of polyclonal antibodies or where the animals are to be maintained as antibody producers for a long period of time, the use of whiffle balls or serum pockets for antibody collection may be considered (Whary *et al.*, 1998).

The nature of the antigen, as well as the intended purpose of the antiserum produced, should be reflected in the choice of the immunization protocol. Adjuvants are used to enhance the immune response. The ideal adjuvant can be characterized as a substance which stimulates high and sustainable antibody titers (even with small quantities of antigen), is efficient in a variety of species, applicable to a broad range of antigens, is easily and reproducibly prepared in an injection mixture, is easily injectable, has low toxicity for the immunized subject, and is not harmful to the investigator. In general, an immunogen should be mixed with an equal volume of adjuvant and emulsified. Emulsification can best be achieved using two Luer-Lok syringes and a locking connector, passing the adjuvant and immunogen back and forth until it becomes paste-like. Sonication using a narrow probe is an alternative method of emulsification; however, care must be taken to avoid overheating by keeping the sonication mixture on ice. Proper preparation of the immunogen/ adjuvant mixture is important as a major cause of immunization failure is due to inappropriate emulsification. Dispersal of the emulsion with an equal volume of 2% Tween 80 reduces the viscosity of the solution for easier injection (Herbert, 1965).

Antibodies presently available for research, diagnostic and therapies are mostly mammalian monoclonal or polyclonal antibodies. The rabbit is the most commonly used animal for the production of polyclonal antibodies as it is easy to handle and to bleed, and for most applications will produce an adequate volume of high-titre, high affinity, antiserum (Stills, 1994). Traditionally, bigger animals such as horses, sheep, pigs, rabbits and guinea pigs were used for the production of polyclonal antibodies, while mice and rats were used for monoclonal antibodies. Now days, most frequently chosen mammals for polyclonal and monoclonal antibody production are rabbits and mice respectively. Both technologies have their advantages but also disadvantages. Major problem of monoclonal antibody production is that some antigens are weakly or not at all immunogenic for mice. In polyclonal antibody production purification of antibodies from mammalian blood has been found low yielding and laborious. Both technologies also involve some steps each of which causes distress to the animals involved: *i*) the immunization itself, *ii*) collecting of blood samples and *iii*) bleeding, which are a prerequisite for antibody preparation (Mojca Narat, 2003).

16.3. Chicken antibodies (IgY) – An alternative Approach

In 1893, Klemperer first demonstrated that the immunization of a hen resulted in the transfer of specific antibodies from the serum to the egg yolk. For over a hundred years there was no scientific application for this knowledge. But when the animal welfare became a matter of serious ethical concern for the scientific community, the results of Klemperer have attracted a great attention, particularly since the 1980s. In the sense of animal welfare, the use of laying hens for antibody production represents a refinement and a reduction in animal use. It is a refinement in that the painful and invasive blood sampling or scarifying are replaced by collecting eggs. It entails a reduction in the number of animals used because the antibodies productivity in laying hens is nearly 18 times greater than that in rabbits (Schade *et al.,* 1996). Furthermore, because of the high yolk antibodies concentration, over 100 mg of antibodies can be obtained from one egg (Akita *et al.,* 1992). Since a laying hen produces approximately 20 eggs per month, 2 g of antibody per month may be obtained from a single laying hen.

Three immunoglobulin classes, which are distinguishable in concentration, structure, and immunochemical function, are found in birds: IgA, IgM, and IgY. The IgA and IgM are similar to mammalian IgA and IgM in molecular weight, structure and electrophoretic mobility. Historically, IgY, the major immunoglobulin class present in avian serum and egg yolk was called IgG, due to its function and serum concentration in comparison with the mammalian IgG. However, it has become clear that this is inappropriate, especially because of fundamental structural differences between IgG and IgY molecules, which will be discussed in more details later. IgY makes up about 75% of the total immunoglobulin pool. The serum concentrations of IgY, IgA, and IgM have been reported to be 5.0, 1.25, and 0.61 mg.ml-1, respectively (Leslie *et al.,* 1973).

Antibodies are transferred from hen to chick via the latent stage of the egg, and play an important role in immunological function for the relatively immuno-incompetent chick to resist various infectious diseases. Serum IgY is selectively transferred from the hen's circulatory system across the oolemma into the maturing oocyte in the ovarian follicle (Rose *et al.,* 1981). The concentrations of IgA (~0.7 mg.ml-1) and IgM (~0.15 mg.ml-1) in egg white are relatively low while that of IgY (8-25 mg.ml-1) in egg yolk is considerably high (Rose *et al.,* 1974).

16.4. Structure and Characteristics of IgY

The main type of immunoglobulin isolated from egg yolk is generally referred to as IgY. Other Ig classes are present, but only in negligible amount. Historically, the low molecular weight Ig found in avian serum was known as IgG, by analogy with its mammalian counterpart. It has become clear, however, that this is inappropriate due to the fundamental structural difference between IgG and IgY. No IgG – like antibody with a heavy y chain of 50,000 Da has been found in the chicken (Warr *et al*., 1995). The data available indicate that IgY is more highly concentrated in yolk than it is in serum (Larsson *et al*., 1993)

Name IgY has been proposed by Leslie and Clem in 1969. The term IgY is originally coined to refer to the larger molecular weight IgY found in egg yolk, but it is now accepted that IgY is the major antibody in both the blood and yolk in concentration of around 10-20 mg/ml.

Fig - The structural differences between mammalian IgG and avian IgY. (Losonczy and Batke, 1997).

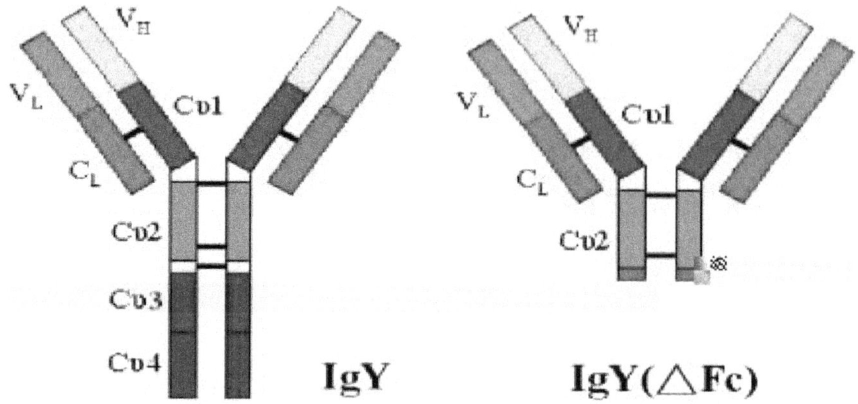

The heavy chain (y) of IgG consists of four domains: the variable domain (V_H) and three constant domains (Cy1, Cy2 and Cy3). The Cy1 domain is separated from Cy2 by a hinge region, which gives considerable flexibility to the Fab fragments. In contrast, the heavy chain of IgY (v) has a molecular weight of 65,000 Da, does not have a hinge region and possesses four constant domains (Cv1-Cv4) in addition to the variable domain. Sequence comparisons between IgG and IgY have shown that the Cy2 and Cy3 domains of IgG are closely related to the Cv3 and Cv4 domains respectively, of IgY, while the equivalent of the Cv2 domain is absent in the IgG, having been replaced by the hinge region (Warr *et al.*, 1995).

The chicken is phylogenetically distant from mammals and, therefore, can be useful for raising polyclonal antibodies to mammalian proteins, and in particular, to intracellular mammalian proteins, as the amino acid sequence of many intracellular proteins tends to be conserved between mammalian species. The product, IgY, is for almost all purposes equivalent to the mammalian IgG class of antibodies. The chicken may be considered as a refinement of technique as polyclonal antibodies can be extracted from the egg yolk, removing the necessity for blood collection. The use of the chicken can also represent a reduction in animal use as chickens produce larger quantities of antibodies than laboratory rodents (Schade *et al.*, 1996; Bollen *et al.*, 1995). Typically, a single egg will contain up to 250mg polyclonal antibodies in the egg yolk (Erhard *et al.*, 2000). In general, chickens are potent antibody producers and their immunological responsiveness is similar to that of mammals. However, it is important to emphasize that the chicken is not suitable for all applications, and appropriate facilities for housing chickens must be available if they are to be used.

16.5. Production and purification of chicken antibodies (IgY)

Specific IgY development and production can be achieved by immunizing laying hens with the target antigen. However, the resulting immune response of the immunized hens cannot be very predictable. Mainly five factors influence this response: the antigen (dose and molecular weight), the type of adjuvant used, the route of application, the immunization frequency, and the interval between immunizations (Schade *et al.*, 1996). Immunization of the chicken results in the formation of specific antibodies which comprise 0.1-10% of IgY in depends on the antigen. To stimulate the immune response of experimental animal, the desired antigen is applied in combination with various adjuvant compounds (Hilgers *et al.*, 1998).

More than 100 years ago, Klemperer (1983) first demonstrated that avian maternal antibodies are transferred from serum to egg yolk in order to protect the developing embryo from potential pathogens but at that time there was no scientific application for this knowledge. However, when animal welfare became a matter of serious ethical concern for the scientific community, the results of Klemperer began to receive more interest, particularly since the 1980s. Since 1996, IgY technology (i.e. the production and use of IgY) has become an internationally accepted practice (Schade, 1996). In 1996, the European Centre for the Validation of Alternative Methods (ECVAM) workshop strongly recommended that IgY should be used as an alternative to mammalian antibodies (Schade, 1997). In 1999, IgY technology was approved as an alternative method for supporting animal welfare by the Veterinary Office of the Swiss Government. In 2005 Schade *et al*, reviewed the production of specific IgY in order to produce specific IgY antibodies, laying hens are immunized with specific foreign pathogens which induce immune responses, including the production of antibodies with activity against these specific disease conditions. These antibodies are then transferred to the egg yolk and deposited in large quantities. Booster immunizations are usually given to ensure continued transfer of antibodies from the hen's serum to the egg yolk. These antibodies are then extracted from the egg yolk and processed to be administered directly to the animal or incorporated into diets (Xiaoyu Li *et al.*, 2015).

IgY Antibodies are then extracted from the egg yolk and processed

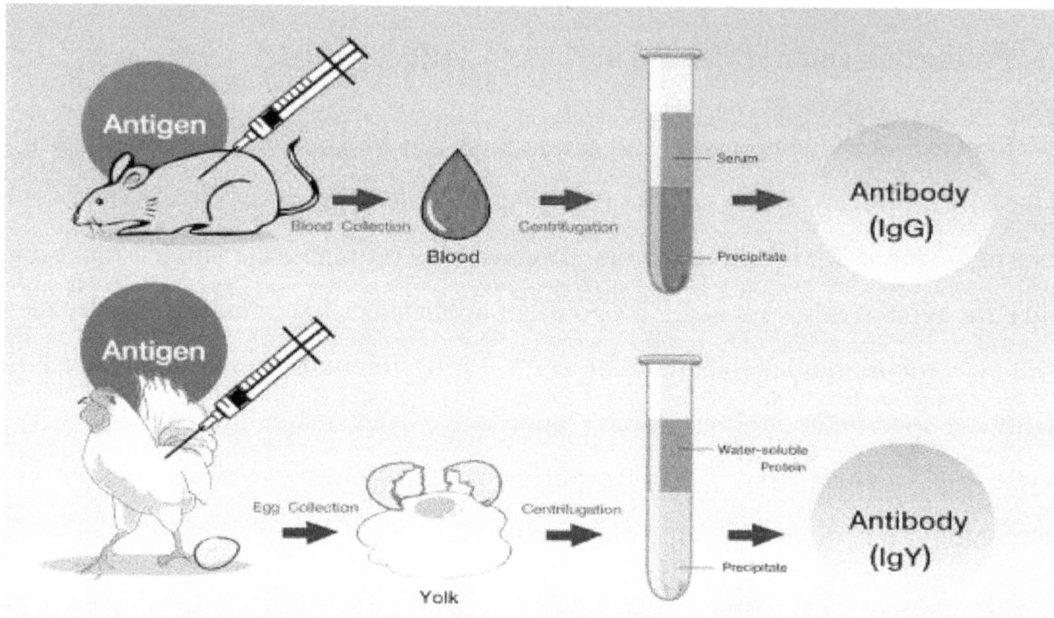

16.6. Advantages of Chicken Antibodies (IgY)

The chicken immune system has been studied for many years, and these studies have contributed substantially to the understanding the fundamental concepts of immunology and the development of different immunoglobulin classes (Carlander *et al.*, 1999). In a report of Sharma, (1997) the use of avian antibodies offers many advantages over mammalian antibodies. Nowadays small quantities of avian antibodies are only used because of the limitation of awareness and handling techniques while using chickens. Traditionally, commercially available polyclonal antibodies have been produced in mammals such as mice, rats, rabbits, sheep, goats, and horses, and are generally obtained from sera after immunization of these animals (Schade *et al.*, 1996). However, these antibodies cannot be prepared on an industrial scale because of the difficulty in obtaining large quantities of blood, and concerns about animal welfare. The use of hybridoma technology has been used for the preparation of monoclonal antibodies; however, it is still far from the successful commercialization of therapeutic monoclonal antibodies due to the expensive cost (Wang and Imanaka, 1995)

References

Akita, E.M and S.Nakai. 1992. Immunoglobulins from egg yolk: Isolation and Purification. *Journal of food science.* **57(3):** 629-634.

Bollen L.S, Hau J. 1995. Chicken eggs in polyclonal antibody production. In:Nevalainen T, Hau J, Sarviharju M, eds. Proceedings of the 10th ICLAS Meeting, Helsinki, Finland. *Scand J Lab Anim Sci Suppl* 1.

Carlander, D., J.Stalberg, A.Larsson.1999. Chicken antibodies: a clinical chemistry perspective. *Ups. J.Med. Sci.* **104**:179-189.

Erchard, M.H., Ozpinar, H., Bilal, T., Abbas, Y., Kutay, C., Wseceli, H. and Stangassinger, M. (2000) The humoral response and the productivity of laying hens kept on the ground or in cages. *Alternatives to Laboratory Animals*, 28:699.

Herbert, W.J. 1965. Multiple emulsions: A new form of mineral-oil adjuvant. Lancet. October **16**:771.

Hilgers, L. A., I.Nicolas, G.Lejeune, E.Dewil, B.Boon.1998. Effect of various adjuvants on secondary immune rsponse in chickens. *Vet. Immunol. Immunopathol.***66**: 159-171.

Larsson, A., R.M.Balow, T.L.Lindahl, and P.O.Forsberg. 1993. Chicken antibodies: taking advantage of evolution. A review. *Poultry Science.* **72**: 1807-1812.

Leslie, G.A. and Martin, L.N. 1973. Studies on the secretory immunologic system of fowl. 3. Serum and secretory IgA of the chicken. *J. Immunol.* **110**:1–9.

Marlies Leenaars, P.P.A., F.M.Coenraad, Hendriksen, A.Wim, De Leeuw, Florina Carat, Philippe Delahaut, René Fischer, Marlies Halder, W. Carey Hanly, Joachim Hartinger, Jann Hau, Erik B. Lindblad, Werner Nicklas, Ingrid M. Outschoorn and Duncan E.S. Stewart-Tull. 1999. The Production of Polyclonal Antibodies in Laboratory Animals. *Alta.* **27**: 79 -109.

Michalek SM, Childers NK.1990. Development and outlook for a caries vaccine. *Crit Rev Oral Biol Med* **1:** 37-54.

Mojca Narat. 2003. Production of Antibodies in Chickens. *Food Technol. Biotechnol.* ***41*** **(3)**: 259 – 267.

Rose, M.E, ORLANS, E. 1981. Immunoglobulins in the egg, embryo and young chick. *In Developmental and Comparative Immunology.* **5:(1),** p. 15–20.

Rose, M.E., E. Orlans, and N.Buttress. 1974. Immunoglobulin classes in the hen's eggs: Their segregation in yolk and white. *Eur. J. Immunol.* **4:** 521: 523.

Schade R. & Hlinak A., 1996. Egg yolk antibodies, state of the art and futurs prospects. *ALTEX*, **13**(1), 5-9.

Smith, D., and Taubman, M. 1995. Experimental immunization of rats with Streptococcus mutans 59-kilodalton glucab-binding protein against dental caries. *Infect. Immun* **64:** 3069-3073.

Stills, H.F. 1994. Polyclonal Antibody Production. In: The Biology of the Laboratory Rabbit, 2nd Edn. (eds. P.J. Manning, D.H. Ringler & C.E. Newcomer). Pp. 435-448. San Diego CA: Academic Press.

Wang, H.Y. and Imanaka, T. (1995) Antibody Expression and Engineering. American Chem. Soc., Washington, DC.

Warr, G.M., K.E. Magor, D.A. Higgens. 1995. IgY: clues to the origins of modern antibodies. *Immunology Today.* **16**: 392-398.

Whary, M.T., Carey, D.D. & Ferguson, F.G. 1998. Reduction in animal numbers required for antisera production using the subcutaneous chamber technique in rabbits. Laboratory Animals **32:**46-54.

Xiao S. Liu· Wen J. Yang· Jin X. He· and Jin Z. Zhao. 2014. Preparation of artificial antigen and egg yolk-derived immunoglobulin (IgY) of florfenicol amine for ELISA assay. *Journal of Environmental Science and Health*, Part B: Pesticides, Food Contaminants, and Agricultural Wastes **49**(2).

HIGHLIGHTS

- There are several chemical agents on the market for oral health, but they all have unfavourable side effects.
- Thus, the hunt for substitute goods and naturally occurring phytochemicals extracted from plants that are utilized as traditional remedies goes on.
- Natural products, primarily derived from plants, and their bio-actively generated chemicals support distinct biological characteristics in inhibiting the growth, adhesion, and colonization of oral bacteria.
- The herbal formulations consist of several different herb combinations. They are all quite promising in treating the oral condition.
- Numerous scientific investigations have shown that the bioactive substances found in plants can have certain unfavourable side effects.
- The WHO advises that, in order to prevent side effects, scientific validation be obtained prior to formulating any herbal remedies.

CHAPTER

17

Herbalism against Dental Caries

Nowadays, in the fight against dental caries, the use of chemical agents such as alcohols, chlorhexidine, and antibiotics (penicillin, ampicillin, etc.) are quite common. However, the treatment methods of dental caries are symptomatic and do not include a preventable approach to bacterial factors that cause dental caries and periodontal diseases. Also, resistance to antibiotics may develop against bacteria in biofilm and this may worsen the prognosis of the disease. To prevent this situation, efforts are underway to develop new anti-infective agents against microorganisms (Projan and Youngman 2002). Western medical/dentistry has achieved limited clinical success in treatment of a variety of oral complaints, such as xerostomia, Apthous ulcer, lichen planus, and Bechet's syndrome. World Health Organization (WHO), American Dental Association (ADA), and the World Dental Federation (FDI) recommend kinds of toothpaste containing fluoride and triclosan. The use of toothpaste containing fluoride and triclosan indeed has benefits. However, excessive use of chemical and synthetic products is harmful. The use of products containing fluoride can cause changes in the intestinal and oral flora and even oral cancer, vomiting, and dental staining. Other chemicals such as chlorhexidine and amine fluoride cause toxic effects. Ethanol, another chemical added to oral products, has been reported to cause cancer (McCullough and Farah, 2008).

Ayurveda is the ancient Indian system of health care and longevity. It involves a holistic view of man, his health, and illness. Ayurvedic treatment is aimed at the patient as an organic whole, and treatment consists of salubrious use of drugs, diets, and certain practices (Sharma, 1979). Currently, *Ayurveda* is widely practiced in the Hindustan peninsula (India and the neighbouring countries) and, in recent years, has attracted much attention in economically developed countries such as those in Europe and in the United States and Japan (Hartzell and Zysk., 1995).

17.1. Phytotherapy

Phytotherapy, which means treatment with plants, is a complementary treatment. All or part of the plants is mixed and used for treatment. During this process, care is taken to preserve the original composition of the plant. When examined in terms of developments in dentistry, phytotherapy is used because of the antimicrobial, anti-inflammatory, analgesic, and sedative properties of plants (Groppo *et al.*, 2008). One of the methods of using plants in the treatment is to obtain essential oils. Essential oils are aromatic liquids with volatile characters and they are obtained from several parts of plants such as leaves, barks, seeds, and roots. Due to their different components which they have, essential oils can show variations of their mechanisms of action. Their usage areas are quite wide due to their antibacterial, insecticidal, and antifungal effects. The first studies that obtained information on the existence of antibacterial properties of essential oils were carried out by Dela Croix in 1881. The data obtained from this study led other studies that used essential oils in medicine in the following centuries. Some essential oils identified by the American Food and Drug Administration have been generally described as generally recognized as safe/GRAS (Generally Recognized as Safe) food additives or taste-smell additives. Essential oils have irritant, antitussive, rubefian, nervinatic, carminative, emmenagogue, diuretic, anthelmintic, antiseptic, anti-inflammatory, antifungal, antioxidant, and antibacterial properties. Essential oils show antibacterial activity against various bacteria, including S. Mutans (Al-Mariri and Safi, 2014).

17.2. Traditional Plant-Based Medicines

Medicinal plants have been used as traditional treatments for numerous human diseases for thousands of years and in many parts of the world. In rural areas of the developing countries, they continue to be used as the primary source of medicine. About 80% of the people in developing countries use traditional medicines for their health care. The natural products derived from medicinal plants have proven to be an abundant source of biologically active compounds, many of which have been the basis for the development of new lead chemicals for pharmaceuticals. With respect to diseases caused by microorganisms, the increasing resistance in many common pathogens to currently used therapeutic agents, such as antibiotics and antiviral agents, has led to renewed interest in the discovery of novel anti-infective compounds. As there are approximately 500 000 plant species occurring worldwide, of which only 1% has been phytochemically investigated, there is great potential for discovering novel bioactive compounds (Kim, 2005).

17.3. Biological Properties of Plants

Traditional knowledge on medicinal plants, used for different health purposes, has attracted much attention among the scientific community due to their effectiveness in the treatment of several diseases (Khan *et al.*, 2012). Medicinal plants are a rich source of bioactive compounds, or bio- nutrients, which may be present in seeds, roots, leaves, flowers, or even in the whole plant, thus assuming themselves as important sources of compounds with characteristics of food additives, flavourings and other valences at an industrial level (Tiwari and Rana, 2005). Bioactive compounds are secondary metabolites that can be classified based on their composition, the pathway by which they are synthesized, or through their chemical structure. A simple classification of bioactive compounds includes three main groups, consisting of phenolic compounds, terpenoids, and alkaloids, which represent about 90% of all secondary metabolites. The minor groups of secondary metabolites include saponins, lipids, carbohydrates, ketones, and others. Currently, phenolic compounds are among the most studied natural products, given their chemical and structural diversity and bioactive properties, which may include antioxidant, antimutagenic, antitumor, antiallergenic, anti-inflammatory, antiviral, antiulcer, antidiarrheal, anthelmintic, antihepatitic, and antiproliferative properties (Carocho *et al.*, 2014). Medicinal plants are composed of a wide range of phenolic compounds with antimicrobial properties that provide protection against aggressive agents. Some of these compounds can deliver sustainable solutions for combating drug-resistant microorganisms. These secondary metabolites are biosynthesized from the shikimate pathway, containing benzene, hydrogen and oxygen rings, the majority of which being flavonoids, the largest and most studied group of compounds in plants (Hassan, 2012). Flavonoids are found to be effective against a wide range of microorganisms, and their antimicrobial activity is thought to be shaped through their ability to form complexes with both extra-cellular and soluble proteins, as well as with bacterial membranes, increasing their permeability and disruption. In addition, these compounds may also act to inhibit the activities of DNA gyrase and _-hydroxyacyl-acyl transport protein dehydratase; for example, catechins belonging to this group exhibit inhibitory activity against both Gram-positive and Gram-negative bacteria (Taylor, *et al.,* 2005). In its turn, apigenin showed inhibitory activity to both GTF and fructosyltransferase proteins of S. mutans without major impact on bacterial viability. Quercetin derivates inhibited S. mutans biofilm production by reducing the synthesis of both water-soluble and insoluble glucans and suppressing several virulence genes. On the other hand, the antimicrobial mechanism by which terpenoid compounds act is not clearly defined, but is attributed to the rupture of microorganism's membrane. Finally, alkaloids, which are biosynthesized from amino acids, such as tyrosine, hold an antimicrobial mechanism attributed to their ability to intercalate with DNA, thereby resulting in impaired cell division and death. The plant-extracted product may exert its antimicrobial activity, not by killing the microorganism itself, but by affecting several key events in the pathogenic process (Sen and Samanta, 2015). The use of herbal extracts and their products on a daily basis is a promising and interesting alternative to synthetic compounds in the control of oral diseases.

17.4. Medicinal Plants against Oral Pathogens

Table – 5- Herbs and its parts used for oral infections

S.l No	Common name	Botanical Name	Parts used	Medicinal properties
1.	Neem	*Azadirachta indica*	Bark and Stem	Antioxidant and Antimicrobial
2.	Garlic	*Allium sativum*	Garlic extract	Antimicrobial
3.	Vine leaf	*Piper beetle*	Leaf extract	Antimicrobial
4.	Rosemary and cinnamon	*Rosemary officinalis*	Woody herb	Antimicrobial
5.	Clove	*Syzygium aromaticum*	Clove oil	Antimicrobial
6.	Walnut	*Juglans regia*	Stem, bark, root, seeds, leaves and oi	Antimicrobial
7.	Spanish Cherry	*Mimusops elengi*	Bark	Antimicrobial
8.	Pomegranate	*Punica granatum*	Leaves, fruits, root, and stem	Decrease the biofilm
9.	Amala, Indian gooseberry,	*Emblica officinalis*	Seed coat	Antimicrobial
10.	Kadukka	*Terminalia chebula*	Seed	Antimicrobial
11.	Miswak tree.	*Salvadora persica*	Roots, and stems	Anti-biofilm and anti-inflammation property
12.	Bloodroot	*Sanguinaria canadensis*	Whole plant	Anti-biofilm and anti-inflammation property
13.	Mempat.	*Cratoxylum formosum*	Gum obtained from Mempat	Reduce dental cavities

14.	Acacia	*Acacia catechu*	heartwood extract	Reduce dental cavities
15.	Paperbark tree	Tea tree oil	Paperbark tree	Oral sanitation
16.	Turmeric	Turmeric	Tubers	Antimicrobial
17.	Aloe vera barbadensis	*Aloe vera*	Gel	Anticancer, antidiabetic, antibiotic properties and reduce teeth biofilm formation

17.5. Different Herbal Formulations

Different herbal formulations are alternative options for prevention and treatment of dental diseases because the product formulations prepared from the herbal sources are safe, effective and economically available as compared to other choices

17.5.1. Herbal chewable tablets: These are an important alternative and convenient to conventional tablets in dental diseases. Such tablets have great and potential merits because of no need of water. It implies that the tablets can be given to the patient at any place in any time. Chewable tablets provide additional advantages for patients to ensure better compliance, to improve the experience and to overcome swallowing difficulties (Hermes-Pharma., 2016). The increasing prevalence of multi drug resistant strains of bacteria and the recent manifestation of strains with abridged susceptibility to antibiotics increases the prevalence of untreatable bacterial infections and poses necessity for searching new infection combating strategies in dental Diseases. Chewable tablets are one of the best remedies available against cariogenic microorganisms (Saraya *et al*., 2008).

17.5.2. Herbal gels: It is defined as semi rigid systems in which movement of the dispersing medium is restricted by an interlacing three-dimensional network of particles from different herbs or solvated macromolecules of the dispersed phase (Goldman, 2001). Herbal gels have better potential as a vehicle to administer drug topically in comparison to ointment, because they are non-sticky, require low energy during formulation, are stable and have aesthetic value (Mohammed Haneefa *et al*., 2012). Herbal gels have several advantages over conventional gels in minimizing side effects and increasing the therapeutic efficacy. Herbal gels with suitable rheological properties can facilitate the absorption of poorly absorbed drug by increasing the contact time of the drug with the skin (Pawar, & Shamkuwar, 2013).

17.5.3. Polyherbal formulations: It refer to formulations in which two or more than two herbs are involved to develop a product to reduce adverse events by enhancing the therapeutic action and reducing the single herbs concentrations. Sometimes, these herbs are combined with mineral preparations (Srivastava *et al.*, 2012) The concept of polyhedral formulation is well-established and documented in the literature of ancient history. Today, a challengeable task is subjected to concern on the development of a stable polyherbal formulation because of the wide diversity of chemical compounds in different medicinal plants (Bhope, *et al.,* 2011). They are compilation of therapeutic entities that are formulated and prepared on the basis of the healing properties of individual ingredients with respect to the condition of sickness. Such herbal constituents with diverse pharmacological activities principally work together in a dynamic way to produce maximum therapeutic benefits with minimum side effects (Barik *et al.,* 2015).

17.5.4. Herbal lollipops: These are sugar-free products made up of licorice extracts using a standard sugar-free candy formula suggested by Dr. John's Candy. The main ingredients of formulations were: hydrogenated starch hydrolysate (HSH) (solidifying agent), citric acid and mint (flavouring agents), FD & C blue #1,2; Red 3, 40; Yellow 5, 6 (coloring agents), and acesulfame potassium (non-caloric sweetener). Licorice extracts (about 7–15 mg) were added to each lollipop to make the uniformity of Glycyrrhizol A concentration. The amounts of licorice extracts are always dependent upon the Glycyrrhizol A concentration in a batch. The lollipop manufacturing comprises various temperatures ranges from maximum 135°C to minimum 65°C for cooking syrup and on the cooling table, respectively. At various temperatures, the thermal stability of Glycyrrhizol A was tested. Then, the extracts of the herbal are added at the particular and appropriate temperatures at which their bioactivities could not be affected. The studies showed that the sugar-free lollipops were safe and their anti-microbial activities against cavity causing bacteria were stable in the formulations intended for delivery. It was also revealed from pilot human studies that a brief application of these lollipops (twice a day for 10 days) led to marked reduction of cavity-causing bacteria in oral cavity among most of the human subjects under study. Therefore, lollipops turn out to be a useful delivery system well accepted by different populations with problems in oral cavity (Chu-hong, *et al.*, (2011).

17.5.5. Herbal Mouthwashes: Mouthwashes are concentrated aqueous solutions of anti-microbial preparations, routinely used in the oral cavity after dilution to counter infections, for cleansing and anti-sepsis as well as refreshing the oral cavity. The health benefits of herbal mouthwashes include: relieving symptoms of gingivitis, canker sores, inflamed gums, sore mouth, inflamed or ulcerated throat, mouth infections, bleeding gums and teeth sensitivity. Mouthwashes are commonly for oral hygiene and in the delivery of active agents to the teeth and gums. The potency of these rinses to influence the plaque formation and to alter the course of gingival inflammation has been reviewed extensively by many researchers. A decoction of the root-bark was suggested as a mouthwash for swollen gums and decoction of the leaves makes an efficacious gargle for swollen gum and ulceration of the mouth and also for bleeding gums (Al-Bayaty, *et al.*, 2004).

17.5.6. Herbal Toothpaste and Toothpowder: Herbal toothpaste consists of a formulation of well-constituted herbs that ensure anti-bacterial and gum tightening properties and provide absolute dental care. It contains natural taste of several ingredients like elaichi (*Elettaria cardamomum*), lavang (*Syzygium aromaticum,* also known as cloves), etc. and helps users in maintaining a fresh mouth for the whole day and also provides ideal protection against dental issues like gum bleeding and sensitivity. Further, the toothpaste is made of uncommon herbs that are safe to use and have great effect on oral hygiene and health (Patki *et al.*, 2013)

17.6. Safety Issues Related to Phytomedicines Used in Dentistry

The clinical studies reviewed above have generally assessed the efficacy of products containing plant-derived products. However, the safety and possible side-effects of such products must also be considered. Indeed, these issues have recently been reviewed in relation to natural products used in dentistry. In agreement with other studies of the clinical use of natural products, these authors have concluded that there is limited information available about the quality, safety and efficacy of herbal products used in dentistry. Given the possibility of adverse interactions between herbal formulations with conventional drugs, caution should be exercised when using herbal medicines and the need for more clinical studies is recommended.

References

Al-Bayaty, F. H., Al-Koubaisi, A. H., Wahid, A. N. A., & Abdulla, M. A., (2004). Effect of mouth wash extracted from *Salvadorapersica*(Miswak) on dental plaque formation, A clinical trial. *Journal of Medicinal Plants Research, 4*(14), 1446–1454.

Al-Mariri A, Safi M. In vitro antibacterial activity of several plant extracts and oils against some gramnegative bacteria. Iran J Medi Sci 2014; 39(1): 36-43.

Barik, C. S., Kanungo, S. K., Tripathy, N. K., Panda, J. R., & Padhi, M. A., (2015). Review on therapeutic potential of polyherbal formulations. *International Journal of Pharmaceutical Science and Drug Research*, *7*(3), 211–228.

Bhope, S. G., Nagore, D. H., Kuber, V. V., Gupta, P. K., & Patil, M. J., (2011). Design and development of a stable polyherbal formulation based on the results of compatibility studies. *Pharmacognosy Research, 3*(2), 122–129.

Carocho, M.; Barreiro, M.F.; Morales, P.; Ferreira, I.C. Adding molecules to food, pros and cons: A review on synthetic and natural food additives. Compr. Rev. Food Sci. Food Saf. **2014**, 13, 377–399.

Chu-hong, H., Jian, H., Randal, E., Xiao-yang, W., Li-na, L., & Yan, T., et al., (2011). Development and evaluation of a safe and effective sugar-free herbal lollipop that kills cavity-causing bacteria. *International Journal of Oral Science*, *3*, 13–20.

Goldman, P., (2001). Herbal medicines today and the roots of modern pharmacology. *Annals of Internal Medicine*, *135*(8), 594–600.

Groppo FC, Bergamaschi CDC, Cogo K, Franz- Montan M, Motta RHL, Andrade, EDD. Use of phytotherapy in dentistry. Phytother. Res. 2008; 22(8):993-998. doi: https://doi.org/10.1002/ptr.2471.

Hartzell JF, Zysk KG. Health, science, and the spirit: Veda and *Ayurveda* in the Western world. J Altern Complement Med. 1995; 1:297–301.

Hassan, B.A.R. Medicinal plants (importance and uses). Pharm. Anal. Acta **2012**, 3, 2153–2435.

Hermes-Pharma., (2016). Chewable Tablets. Hermes Pharma, Germany.

Khan, R.; Adil, M.; Danishuddin, M.; Verma, P.K.; Khan, A.U. In vitro and in vivo inhibition of Streptococcus mutans biofilm by Trachyspermum ammi seeds: An approach of alternative medicine. Phytomedicine **2012**, 19, 747–755.

Kim, H.-S. "Do not put too much value on conventional medicines," *Journal of Ethnopharmacology*, 2005. vol. 100, no. 1-2, pp. 37–39.

Mattick CR. Stomatology- an intriguing blend of traditional Chinese medicine and Western style dentistry. Br Dent J. 1995; 178:350–3.

McClure FJ, Hewitt WL. The relation of penicillin to induced rat dental caries and oral L. acidophilus. J. Dent. Res. 1946; 25(6): 441-443.

McCullough, MJ, Farah CS. The role of alcohol in oral carcinogenesis with particular reference to alcoholcontaining mouthwashes. Aust. Dent. J. 2008; 53(4):302–305. doi: https://doi.org/10.1111/j.1834- 7819.2008.00070.x.

Mohammed Haneefa, K. P., Mohanta, G. P., & Nayar, C., (2012). Formulation and Evaluation of Herbal Gel of Basellaalba for wound healing activity. *Journal of Pharmacological Science and Research*, *4*(1), 1642–1648.

Patki, P. S., Mazumdar, M., Majumdar, S., & Chatterjee, A., (2013). Evaluation of the safety and efficacy of complete care herbal toothpaste in controlling dental plaque, gingival bleeding and periodontal diseases. *Journal of Homeopathy & Ayurvedic Medicine. 2*, 124.

Pawar, D. P., & Shamkuwar, P. B., (2013). Formulation and evaluation of herbal gel containing lantana camara leaves extract. *Asian Journal of Pharmaceutical and Clinical Research, 6*(3), 122–124.

Projan SJ, Youngman PJ. Antimicrobials: New solutions badly needed. Curr. Opin. Microbiol. 2002; 5(5): 463–465. doi: https://doi.org/10.1016/s1369- 5274(02)00364-8.

Saraya, S., Kanta, I., Sarisuta, N., Temsiririrkkul, R., Suvathi, Y., & Samranri K., et al., (2008). Development of Guava Extract Chewable Tablets for Anticariogenic Activity against streptococcus Mutans. *Mahidol University Journal of Pharmaceutical Sciences*, *35*(1-4), 18–23.

Sen, T.; Samanta, S.K. Medicinal plants, human health and biodiversity: A broad review. Adv. Biochem. Eng. Biotechnol. **2015**, 147, 59–110.

Sharma S, editor. Realms of Ayurveda. New Delhi: Arnold- Heineman; 1979.

Srivastava, S., Lal, V. K., & Pant, K. K., (2012). Polyherbal formulations based on Indian medicinal plants as antidiabetic phytotherapeutics. *Phytopharmacology*, *2*(1), 1–15.

Taylor, P.W.; Hamilton-Miller, J.M.T.; Stapleton, P.D. Antimicrobial properties of green tea catechins. Food Sci. Technol. Bull. Funct. Foods **2005**, 2, 71–81.

Tiwari, R.; Rana, C. Plant secondary metabolites: A review. Int. J. Eng. Res. Gen. Sci. **2015**, 3, 661–670.

List of Abbreviations

AAPD - American Academy of Paediatric Dentistry

AAPD - American Academy of Paediatrics

AD - Alzheimer's Disease

ADA - American Dental Association

AFDA - American Food and Drug Administration

AHA - American Heart Association

APOE - Apolipoprotein E

ART - Atraumatic Caries Removal

CDS – Centre for Disease Control

CHD - Congenital Heart Abnormalities

DCI - Dental Council of *India*

ECC - Early Childhood Caries

ESC - European Society of Cardiology

FDI - World Dental Federation

GDB - Global Disease Burden

GRAS - Generally Recognized as Safe

IE - Infective Endocarditis

NHANES - National Health and Nutrition Examination Survey

SGR – Surgeons General Report

SSB – Sugar sweetened Beverages

WHO - World Health Organization

www.ingramcontent.com/pod-product-compliance
Ingram Content Group UK Ltd.
Pitfield, Milton Keynes, MK11 3LW, UK
UKHW060020200726
13845UKWH00057B/1089

9 788197 863653